EMOTIONAL ASPECTS OF HEART DISEASE

Harold Geist, Ph.D. *

*Lecturer in Psychology, San Francisco State University, San Francisco, California and Staff, Everett Gladman Memorial Hospital, Oakland, California

Library of Congress Catalog Card No. 76-16319

391 Willets Road
Roslyn Heights, New York 11577

Manufactured in the United States of America

TABLE OF CONTENTS

To: Marti

ACKNOWLEDGEMENTS

A several year project of this kind requires the cooperation of many people. First, I would like to thank the research assistants, C. Devon Heck, Marianne Minor, and Peter Zellinger who administered and scored the psychological tests and skillfully interviewed cardiac patients. The collation of the data was patiently and accurately done by Susan Baar who also typed much of the manuscript. To the cardiologists who diagnosed the patients, each in his own cardiology unit, Walter Stullman, M.D., at Highland Hospital in Oakland, California and Robin Saphir M.D., at Herrick Memorial Hospital in Berkeley, California, a special note of gratitude for their assistance in classifying various kinds of cardiac patients and giving each a specific diagnosis or diagnoses. Several physicians in private practice, notably Jerome Kaufman, M.D. and Helen Myers, M.D. gave special impetus to the project by allowing us to interview and test their cardiac patients. Arthur Gladman, M.D., Director of Gladman Psychiatric Hospital, Clinic and Foundation, was especially encouraging and helpful from the inception of the research. Donald Walters, M.D. reviewed the manuscript and gave useful suggestions. James Cameron, Ph.D. was especially helpful in the formulation of the cluster analysis. Finally, my deepest thanks goes to the cardiac patients, many of them quite ill, who gave of their time and effort so that they and others similarly afflicted might be helped.

Harold Geist

PREFACE

The general public was surprised when in March of 1974 the idea was postulated that "heart attacks" were caused by the personality and behavior of the people who experienced them. The work of Rosenman and Friedman, however, had previously signalled to the scientific community that behavior dynamics was an important aspect in the etiology of coronary artery disease. It may come as a greater surprise that within the large spectrum of heart disease, of which coronary artery disease is only one segment, there are differences in behavior of those people afflicted. In the following pages, you will see that people with arteriosclerotic heart disease have different dynamics from those with valvular diseases, hypertensive vascular disease, or disturbances of conduction. Perhaps an understanding of these dynamics may help prevent *all* kinds of heart disease and help physicians in treating these ailments.

FOREWORD

Over the past century the contributions of medical science have made possible the virtual eradication of infectious diseases and have contributed greatly to the understanding and management of many other types of illnesses. Those diseases most in need of study fall under the heading of psychophysiological, or more popularly, psychosomatic diseases. These are the stress-related diseases of aging.

I hope that Doctor Geist's pioneering work on the emotional aspects of heart disease will spur more research into the many unexplored areas of psychosomatic illness.

Arthur E. Gladman, M.D.
Director, Everett Gladman
Memorial Foundation, Hospital
and Clinic
Oakland, California

Chapter One

THE PROBLEM

Disease of the heart is one of America's greatest national problems. It is estimated that 10-12 million Americans suffer from the more serious diseases of the heart and circulation, while 15 million are afflicted with less serious diseases. The economic toll of cardiovascular disability is overwhelming. Almost 700,000 man-years are lost in industry each year because of cardiovascular disabilities. This loss in man-years is equivalent to almost three billion dollars in earnings by those disabled by heart disease, and 450 million in federal income tax revenue. With this money the federal government could have provided 60,000 fully equipped high schools. Industrial absenteeism in the United States resulting from cardiovascular disease and its complications is surpassed in incidence only by respiratory disease. In a worldwide survey it was found that one out of every six cardiac patients fails to return to work for psychological reasons, even after being told by his physician that he is in good health. If this is so, then about 200,000 people are so affected since about a million and a half people in this country suffer myocardial infarction each year—with about one million deaths.

CLASSIFICATION OF HEART DISEASE

Heart disease has so many manifestations; it is one of the few illnesses which presents unusual obstacles to orderly classification. However, the New York Heart

Association developed a relatively simple classification of the functional status of cardiac patients which is now accepted and used by a wide variety of clinicians. Patients are divided into four classes:

Class I	Patients who have organic heart disease, but can perform all customary activities without significant symptoms.
Class II	Patients who have symptoms when performing ordinary, moderately strenuous activities; they tolerate less than ordinary activities well and are comfortable at rest.
Class III	Patients who are restricted by symptoms so that less than ordinary activities, even minor ones, produce discomfort; they are comfortable at rest.
Class IV	Patients who can perform no physical activities without some discomfort and usually have symptoms at rest as well.

This is a very subjective classification made primarily from what the patient tells the physician. It may or may not be reliable.

Selzer, on the other hand, has devised what he calls a "therapeutic" classification of heart disease and has divided this into the following:

A. Patients are permitted to undertake unlimited physical effort.
B. Patients' only restriction concerns avoidance of severe or competitive effort.
C. Patients' ordinary physical activities are moderately restricted and strenuous activities eliminated altogether.
D. Patients are permitted to engage only in minor activities.

E. Patients are placed on a rest regimen, confined to bed or chair.

These represent a functional classification insofar as activity is concerned. However, the best classification seems to be in the areas of etiology and structural abnormalities supplemented by physiological disorders. These are determined by cardiac catheterization techniques.*

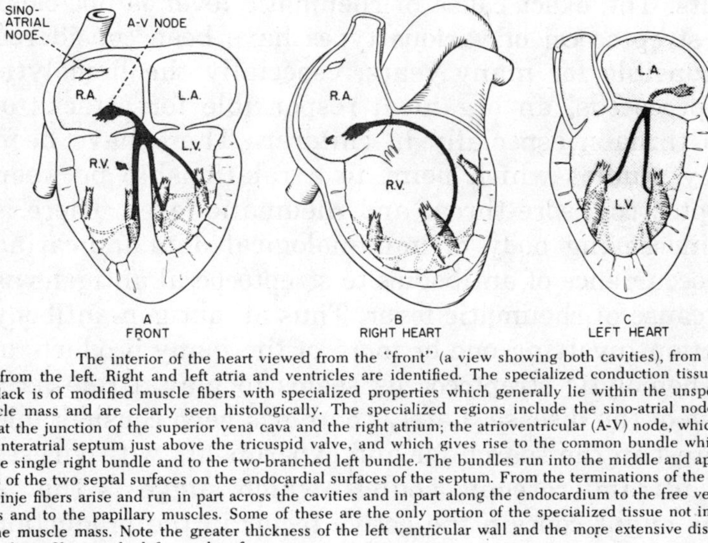

The interior of the heart viewed from the "front" (a view showing both cavities), from the right and from the left. Right and left atria and ventricles are identified. The specialized conduction tissue shown in black is of modified muscle fibers with specialized properties which generally lie within the unspecialized muscle mass and are clearly seen histologically. The specialized regions include the sino-atrial node, which lies at the junction of the superior vena cava and the right atrium; the atrioventricular (A-V) node, which lies in the interatrial septum just above the tricuspid valve, and which gives rise to the common bundle which leads to the single right bundle and to the two-branched left bundle. The bundles run into the middle and apical portions of the two septal surfaces on the endocardial surfaces of the septum. From the terminations of the bundles, Purkinje fibers arise and run in part across the cavities and in part along the endocardium to the free ventricular walls and to the papillary muscles. Some of these are the only portion of the specialized tissue not imbedded in the muscle mass. Note the greater thickness of the left ventricular wall and the more extensive distribution of Purkinje fibers to the left septal surface.

Reprinted from "Physiology and Biophysics, Circulation, Respiration and Fluid Balance" by Howell and Fulton (20th edition, 1974, Chapter 7, page 103, with the permission of W. B. Saunders Co., Philadelphia, Pa.

* The classification here is one recommended by Selzer, Arthur; The Heart—Its Function in Health and Disease, University of California Press, 1966.

I Rheumatic Carditis

The name rheumatic fever hints at this disease occurring because of inflammation of the joints. It is characterized by occurrence of inflammatory lesions in many parts of the body, notably the heart, blood vessels, and joints. Climatic conditions, and to a great extent heredity, have been thought to be important controlling factors. It is particularly a disease of the young, crippling and killing many youths and young adults. The exact cause of rheumatic fever is not clear but streptococci of various types have been considered responsible for many years, especially the hemolytic streptococcus, an organism responsible for attacks of sore throats, especially in children. There have been many studies which point to a relationship between streptococcal sore throat and rheumatic fever. There is an increasing body of immunological data indicating the occurrence of antibodies to streptococcal antigens as the cause of rheumatic fever. Thus an antigen-antibody reaction involving one or more of the many products of the hemolytic streptococcus seems to play a role as a cause of the disease. Lately there has been considerable interest in the search for and experiments with viruses and ultramicroscopic bodies—which suggests that a virus might contain the active factor in the production of rheumatic infection, but there is no experimental evidence for this assumption.

The geographical distribution of rheumatic fever is rather interesting. In the United States, the New England, North Atlantic, and Rocky Mountain states have the highest incidence; next comes the Great Lakes Region, and the South and Far West with the lowest incidence. One of the problems in recording the incidence of rheumatic fever in many communities is the difficulty of diagnosis. Susceptibility to rheumatic fever ascends to age 4, reaches its peak at 10 and declines sharply after the age of 20. It runs in families but is not inherited according to Mendelian laws, and seems to be more prevalent in families of lower socioeconomic status.

The symptoms of rheumatic fever are rather diverse but include fever, pain arising from inflammation of the joints, abdominal pain, skin changes and St. Vitus Dance (Chorea). There is also loss of appetite, loss of weight, weakness and fatigability. There is involvement of all three layers of the heart (known as pancarditis), endocardium, myocardium, and pericardium transient rashes or small nodules under the skin, and painful swelling of the joints. Early in the disease there is a destruction of the myocardium resulting in an enlargement of the heart. Then Aschoff bodies which are inflammatory cells in the heart tissues, finally heal. The valves may then become thickened and function faultily. Thus, because it is in the healing process that the valves become affected, it may be difficult to predict whether chronic heart disease will develop. Very often pneumonia will set in but it usually leaves no after effects.

There is no specific diagnostic laboratory test for rheumatic heart disease. Some have used sedimentation rate and the antistreptolysin titer, neither of which is quite satisfactory. An abnormal reading in the sedimentation rate means simply that there is an abnormality in constituents of the blood serum found in many diseases. The elevation of antistreptolysin titer is characteristic of strep sore throat as well as rheumatic fever.

II. Endocarditis

Endocarditis is an inflammation of the endocardium, the membrane lining the cavities of the heart. Bacterial endocarditis is caused by the lodging of bacteria upon the endocardium. Bacterial endocarditis is divided into two types, acute and subacute.

Acute Endocarditis: Acute Endocarditis is caused by highly destructive (virulent) bacteria which attack the heart valves secondarily. The symptoms are the same as any severe infection with septicemia or blood infection. Acute bacterial endocarditis progresses almost invariably in rapid strides to a fatal termination in days or weeks.

Subacute Bacterial Endocarditis: This disease is an illness of the heart itself and infection of the endocardium and the heart valves occur almost exclusively on areas showing previous damage. The most common organism invading the endocardium in the subacute type of endocarditis is the streptococcus viridans, an organism of low virulence which turns green when cultured in a topical media. Slow and gradual destruction of the heart valves may cause them to be inefficient, and openings in these valves result in murmurs. The bacteria produce vegetations which may in turn produce emboli. With the recent introduction of all kinds of antibiotics, subacute bacterial endocarditis is now 90% curable.

III. Acute Myocarditis

Myocarditis is an inflammation of the heart muscle. It used to be thought that myocarditis was due to either acute rheumatic fever or diptheria. However, abnormalities of cardiac functions due to infections such as virus infections, parotitis (mumps), viral hepatitis, infectious mononucleosis and other septic bloodstream infections (bacterial and fungal) can also cause myocarditis. Diagnosis is usually made by the electrocardiogram and X-ray, the latter showing an enlargement of the heart.

IV. Acute Pericarditis

Pericarditis is an inflammation of the pericardium or outer lining of the heart. It can be caused by a variety of conditions. Viruses, tuberculosis and various bacteria can invade the pericardium. It can also occur as a complication of involvement of other parts of the heart, in rheumatic fever or myocardial infarction. Chronic pericarditis can result from uremic poisoning, a disease of the kidneys. Pericarditis can also occur as the result of a tumor, or of rheumatoid arthritis, periarteritis nodosa and lupus. Pericarditis occurs in two forms—dry pericarditis and pericarditis with effusion. Benign idiopathic pericarditis, a form occurring in relatively young persons, is especially important in our discussion since the difference in diagnosis between it and coronary occlusion which causes a "heart attack," may be difficult. Another form of pericarditis of interest here is the "allergic" pericarditis related to general hypersensitivity to pollens, foods, various chemical compounds, etc.

V. Atherosclerosis and Coronary Disease

Atherosclerosis is a disease where fat-containing materials are deposited beneath the internal surfaces of the blood vessels. The coronary arteries supplying blood to the heart are particularly vulnerable to disturbances of circulation produced by atherosclerosis. It is one of the most important problems in the whole medical-psychiatric-health fields today. Post mortem examinations indicate that in more than 50% of North Americans who die before the age of 50, atheromatous plaques are demonstrable, and among those who die after the age of 75, more than 90% are moderately affected. Heredity (Jewish people have a relatively high incidence), and age (women in the younger age group suffer relatively little and those in the older age group a great deal) seem to be potent influences. It is speculated that there is something in the chemical composition of the plasma of man which makes him more vulnerable than other species. The yellow spots and streaks seen on the internal surface of the blood vessels are deposits of various fatty substances. It is hypothesized that atherosclerosis is either a disturbance of fat metabolism or that of intravascular blood clotting. Selzer (1) believes that, in part, both are correct. In general, those who show low levels of fatty substances in the blood also show low levels of atherosclerosis; those with a high fat content develop atherosclerosis. The usual way to measure fat content is by blood cholesterol.* Hypertension is a very powerful factor accelerating the formation of atherosclerosis. Obesity is also a factor in the formation of

* The mechanisms of the manifestation of cholesterol and fatty diet are related to this study since fat intake was one of the questions on the questionnaire. The two chief providers of blood cholesterol are the liver and intestines. In the liver, various proteins are joined to the cholesterol molecule. In the intestine, the cholesterol is dissolved in fat, phospholipid and a protein similar to the alpha lipoprotein. This "ball" is known as a chylomicron. These chylomicrons enter the bloodstream within minutes after eating a fat and cholesterol containing meal. Some of the chylomicrons may precipitate out

atherosclerosis but the exact relationship is not known; the incidence of heart disease in general is 50% higher in overweight persons than those with normal weight. It is estimated that atherosclerosis of the coronary arteries is responsible for 25-40% of all heart disease. Atherosclerosis is the most frequent cause of cerebral thrombosis and hemmorhage in general, since hemmorhage is thought to result from the rupture of an atherosclerotic vessel in the presence of high blood pressure.

VI. Coronary Artery Disease

The coronary arteries, the first peripheral branches given off by the aorta, are subject to narrowing and complete obstruction due to atheromatosis leading to arteriosclerosis. The chief effect of these lesions is to interfere with coronary blood flow and prevent an adequate blood supply to the myocardium. Atherosclerosis is not the only cause of occlusion of the coronary arteries but is the cause in a great majority of cases. Cardiac pain is generally regarded as the result of an insufficient supply of blood to meet the requirements of the myocardium. "Heart attack" refers to damage to a portion of the heart muscle and quite often "coronary thrombosis" and coronary occlusion are used interchangeably with myocardial infarction, although the latter is the more correct. Although occlusion of one coronary artery may cause a serious deficiency of blood

in the blood and may enter the lining wall of an artery for long periods of time. Physicians and scientists who study this phenomenon think that it is the chylomicrons which are cholesterol rich that come from fatty food and tend to adhere to the arterial walls and ultimately are the cause of heart attacks.

flow to the myocardium, the results may be mitigated by the collateral circulation which can cushion the effect of a heart attack where 20% of the myocardium is damaged. Angina pectoris is a syndrome consisting of chest pains radiating to the shoulders and inner aspects of the arms, precipitated by exertion, emotion, or other states in which the work of the heart is increased. However, there are factors other than exercise which may produce increased demands on the coronary circulation, such as a drop in blood pressure. Men are affected about five times as often as women. It is most frequent at the 6th or 7th decade. In those cases which appear in the 30's and 40's, heredity plays a very important part. The emotional etiology of angina will be discussed in detail in a subsequent chapter. Very often "neurocirculatory asthenia" is confused with angina pectoris. The differences in the two is that "neurocirculatory asthenia" is a pain over long periods of time and unrelated to effort. The pain is over the heart or stomach rather than under the breastbone, and tends to be more neurotically induced.

The cause of coronary artery disease is highly unpredictable. Mild attacks occurring occasionally may characterize an insidious onset. In some patients the symptoms are not slowly progressive but proceed in step-like gradations remaining stationary for many months or years, becoming suddenly more intense and then remaining stationary. In practically all patients, for long periods of time the attacks are induced with regularity by practically the same amount of effort. In all patients the clinical course may be abruptly altered by such unpredictable catastrophic events as acute myocardial infarction, cardiac standstill and even death. The prognosis of myocardial infarction is unpredictable but may provide certain guidelines for estimating whether the prognosis is favorable or not. Treatment of the acute episode in the course of coronary disease (myocardial infarction) is effective in reducing or eliminating certain complications, and therefore in saving lives. The treatment is usually threefold—rest, providing collateral circulation to undamaged heart muscles to take over the function of the entire heart, and preventing complications. The principle guideline is that the patient live within the limits set by his pain.

VII. Hypertension

Hypertension may be defined simply as an abnormal elevation of the blood pressure. An elevated blood pressure may result from a variety of causes which may or may not be of clinical significance. Hypertensive disease as opposed to simple blood pressure elevation is characterized by: 1) A sustained elevation of blood pressure; 2) The appearance of cardiac, renal, retinal, and cerebral vascular complications. Hypertensive disease occurs in about 5% of the adult population.

It has been shown that tension is definitely a cause of hypertension. This will be discussed later on when we consider the psychiatric and psychological aspects of heart disease. There is usually no sharp dividing line between normal and high blood pressure, since individual variations are so great. There seems to be a familial diathesis. Selzer (2) divided hypertension into the following areas 1) Hypertension with a known cause in which cure is possible by removing its cause; 2) Hypertension with a known cause but no cure; 3) Hypertension with unknown origin ("essential hypertension"). Essential hypertension is the most common variety of elevation of blood pressure. There are two forms which are recognized, benign hypertension and malignant hypertension. Hypertension of any type can lead to enlargement of the left ventricle and heart failure, can accelerate the atherosclerotic process in the arteries, can lead to serious complications in the eyes and kidneys, and hemmorhages within the brain or spinal cord (stroke). Benign hypertension can persist for many years, permitting an active and asymptomatic life for long periods of time, and is controllable by medication. Malignant hypertension, on the other hand, is a very serious disease and may lead to disability or death within a very short period of time. Malignant hypertension occurs in young people, often in their 30's.

Insofar as treatment is concerned, in this illness, the most important therapeutic principle is the prevention of anxiety in the patient over his blood pressure. It is here that the principle of "learned anxiety" is very important, since any anxiety exhibited by the physician is immediately transmitted to the patient. Thus, most cardiologists today believe that the patient should be permitted to lead a "normal" life if complications are not indicated. In some cases, cutting a nerve (sympathectomy) has produced genuine reversal of hypertension. Drugs which act as ganglionic blockers, hydralozine, certain tranquilizers, DOPA, and derivatives of chlorthiozide have been beneficial in specific cases.

VALVULAR DISEASES

Any one of the four valves of the heart can be affected for a variety of reasons. The term "chronic valvular heart disease" includes any permanent organic deformity of one or more of the cardiac valves. The cardiac valves can be altered in two ways: First, the valve may be incapable of opening completely so that there is a narrowing of the orifice, or it will not close completely, causing an insufficient amount of blood going into the next chamber, and a backing up of blood in the next chamber. Three of the valves, the mitral, aortic, and tricuspid are subject to acquired malformations while the pulmonary valve anomalies are almost always defective from birth. Most valvular diseases are rheumatic in origin.

Mitral disease is the most common form of chronic valvular disease and comprises well over half of all valvular heart disease. Most adult patients with disability of the mitral valve have mitral stenosis, a narrowing of the orifice of the mitral valve. When the obstruction exceeds one half of the orifice, a "murmur" appears—a coarse rumbling sound of low pitch heard near the cardiac apex. In many patients with mitral stenosis there is a clicking or snapping sound heard at the beginning of the murmur. In recent years the whole field of valvular heart disease has undergone drastic changes because of the possibility of surgical correction of faulty valves. Mitral insufficiency can be diagnosed by cardiac catheterization and is rheumatic in origin. Surgical treatment of mitral insufficiency requires open heart surgery with considerable risk to life.

AORTIC STENOSIS

Aortic stenosis is somewhat similar to mitral stenosis but is due to the deposition of calcium on the aortic valve. It is chiefly a disease of older men, being more frequent in patients past 50 years of age than in younger persons. The deposits result in a build-up of resistance to the ejection of blood from the left ventricle to the aorta. There is an undersupply of blood to the heart and with the increased demands for coronary flow, the lower pressure in the aorta cannot drive sufficient blood into the coronary circulation to meet the demand. The symptoms are very much the same as angina pectoris—chest pains, dizziness, and loss of consciousness. Sometimes there are epileptiform seizures, a harsh aortic systolic murmur, a systolic thrill, a decreased pulse pressure, and a faint, slowly rising pulse. At the present time the chief treatment is by open heart surgery, and the replacement of the natural valve with an artificial valve.

AORTIC INSUFFICIENCY

Incompetence of the aortic valve is known as aortic insufficiency and may be caused by rheumatic involvement, subacute bacterial endocarditis, a blow on the chest, or less frequently, congenital syphilis. The diagnosis is made by a tell-tale heart murmur, poor arterial pulse and a low level of diastolic pressure. As in stenosis, treatment consists of placing a plastic valve in place of the incompetent one.

TRICUSPID STENOSIS AND INSUFFICIENCY

Almost all cases of stenosis of the tricuspid valve are of rheumatic origin. Rheumatic damage to the tricuspid valve commonly produces stenosis and insufficiency of that valve. Tricuspid disease rarely occurs as an isolated lesion; usually a stenosis of the mitral valve is associated with it and aortic valve involement is found in one-third of the cases. Tricuspid stenosis causes an increased work load on the right ventricle and a damming of blood in the right atrium and the veins entering it. Stenosis and insufficiency of the tricuspid valve may cause edema and liver congestion. Tricuspid disease is usually diagnosed by observation of veins in the neck, and treatment is directed at correction of heart failure, and in some cases heart surgery.

CONGENITAL DEFECTS

Congenital heart defects comprise those conditions in which there are abnormalities in the anatomic structure of the heart or great vessels due to abnormal development during embryonic life. The total incidence is about one to two percent of all organic heart disease in all age groups. It is estimated that the incidence of hereditary types of congenital heart disease runs between one and two percent. Rubella, nutritional deficiencies, reduced oxygen content, drugs, and various infectious illness (especially viral diseases) may cause congenital heart malformations. The chief effects of these abnormalities are: a) shunting of the blood between two sides of the circulation; b) obstruction of the normal flow of blood. The classification of congenital heart disease is a complex one, but the following are the most common.

Group I—Non Cyanotic Abnormalities: These are conditions where there is no communication between the two circulations. This may occur in dextrocardia; the heart is on the right side of the chest with the apex pointing to the right. In this classification there are also abnormalities of the aortic arch—coarctation or narrowing of the descending aorta beyond the exit of the subclavian artery. There are two types, the "infantile," a narrowing of a considerable portion of the aortic arch as a result of which the child usually dies early; and the "adult type" in which there is localized narrowing of the aorta near the origin of the subclavian artery. Children with coarctation of the aorta may have high blood pressure from infancy. Surgery is the treatment of choice for this abnormality. Sometimes the bicuspid aortic valves undergo thickening, fibrosis, and scarring causing an acyanotic congenital heart condition. Of the four valves, the pulmonary valve is the one, which if diseased, is almost always affected from birth. Narrowing of the pulmonary artery occurs in two forms. In "valvular stenosis" the fused valves form a dome-shaped projection with a central opening. In "infundibular stenosis" there is a narrowing of varying degrees of the outflow area of the right ventricle. Diagnosis is by cardiac catheterization. Abnormalities of the pulmonary veins which bring blood back to the lung will vary in effect depending on the number of pulmonary veins entering the wrong chambers. When all four veins are involved, congestive heart failure and death usually occur in infancy. Patent ductus stenosis or failure of closure of the ductus arteriosus may cause a systolic and diastolic murmur associated with a "thrill" in the pulmonic area. Elimination of the shunt is usually by surgery. Ventricular septal defects are of two types, small and large. Small ventricular septal defects represent a wide range of conditions varying from mild to serious heart lesions. Ventricular septal defects associated with shunts which affect less then fifty percent of the output of the left ventricle alter the circulation very little. These patients have no symptoms and quite often lead normal lives. Those with ventricular septal defects of more than fifty percent of the left ventricular output often develop cardiac enlargement and may become disabled by symptoms and proceed into heart failure. Those patients with large ventricular septal defects result in pulmonary high blood pressure. Pulmonary hypertension may be high flow or high resistance. Children with high flow pulmonary hypertension resulting from large ventricular septal defect can be operated on, and if they survive the first year of life, may live normally thereafter. The large ventricular septal defects develop pulmonary high blood pressure. Pulmonary hypertension may produce such a high blood pressure through the pulmonary system that it may cause a reversal in the shunt, producing cyanosis which may develop very gradually during life. Surgical treatment of large ventricular defects is moderately successful.

CYANOTIC HEART DISEASE

The most common anomaly in this classification is the Tetrology of Fallot, which is a large ventricular septal defect with pulmonary stenosis. The obstruction of the blood flow from the right ventricle to the pulmonary artery may occur right at the pulmonary valve or underneath it. When obstruction is severe, we get a great deal of cyanosis and a condition known as "blue baby," in which the infant may vary from a slight bluish tinge to deep blue in the entire body. The treatment of choice is surgical intervention known as the Blalock-Taussig procedure. Open heart surgery in general is the treatment of choice, preceded by cardiac catheterization for diagnostic purposes.

There are other congenital malformations of the heart but since those afflicted rarely survive to adult life, these will not be discussed here.

The stimulus which initiates the heart beat arises in the sinus node (SA) which is in the right atrium. This spreads in a radial fashion over the atria and there induces the contraction. After arriving at the atrioventricular (AV) node, which is beneath the endocardium of the right atrium, it proceeds down the atrioventricular bundle and then goes over the right and left branches in the ventricular septum and is then distributed by the Purkinje's fibers to the ventricular muscle—which results in the synchronous contraction of the two ventricles. The activity of the sinus node is affected by the vagus and the accelerator nerves which control the rhythm of the heart. The heart beat is controlled by the sinoatrial node and is called the normal or sinus rhythm. Normal individuals have a regular sequence of heart action of about 70 beats per minute when resting. When the sinus discharge is irregular, this is called an arrhythmia. When the heart rate exceeds 100 beats per minute this is called tachycardia. A rate below 60 beats per minute is a bradycardia. Tachycardia may be caused by a physiological response to exercising, eating, excitement and fear. It also occurs in neurocirculatory asthenia, anemia, hyperthyroidism, rheumatic carditis, myocardial infarction and heart failure. Bradycardia occurs during sleep. It may be associated with malnutrition, jaundice, and increased intracranial pressure. Single beats which are associated with abnormal impulse formation may take their origin in the atrium, the AV node, or the conducting systems within the ventricles, and are known as ectopic beats or extrasystoles. They are caused by temporary irritability in the original focus and appear before the anticipated next beat of the SA node, and are known as premature beats. Ectopic tachycardia is an abnormality of cardiac rhythm consisting of rapid heart beat originating in an overactive or irritable atrial or nodal focus or a ventricular focus. They are usually temporary with sudden onset and sudden termination. Atrial flutter is a partial disorganization of the beat of the atrium at an average rate of about 300 per minute. Atrial fibrillation is a total disorganization of rhythm occurring in specific kinds of heart disease such as abnormalities of the mitral valve, but occasionally is found in individuals who have no detectable cardiac disease. Ventricular flutter and fibrillation are anomalies similar to that of the atrium, but are in the ventricle and usually produce cardiac arrest leading to death. It is particularly common in coronary heart disease.

HEART BLOCKS

Delays of conduction occurring between the atrium and ventricles are caused by a slowing of the transit of impulses through the AV node. This block may be transient, frequent, recurrent, or may occur over long periods of time. It may be caused by certain drugs or take place in the course of some acute illness involving the heart. When the sinus node is quiescent for a few seconds, syncope (fainting) may result. Mild delayed atrioventricular conduction is known as second degree heart block. Here some impulses never reach the ventricle, producing "dropped beats." This is known as the Wenkenbach phenomenon. When total interruption occurs, this is a complete heart block. Failure of the ventricular pacemaker causes loss of consciousness and is known as cardiac syncope or Stokes-Adams attack, or a loss of consciousness. Anything over four minutes is fatal. Complete block is most common in arteriosclerotic heart disease with or without myocardial infarction in some types of congenital heart disease and in rheumatic carditis.

CHRONIC MYOCARDIAL DISEASES

Chronic myocarditis may result from acute involvement of the myocardium or an inflammatory disease without an acute stage. It develops as a gradual enlargement of the heart associated with decrease in the patient's capabilities to perform work and leads to myocardial insufficiency and heart failure. Various metabolic illnesses such amyloidosis and glycogen storage disease may affect the myocardium. Myxoma, a kind of tumor of the atrium, may obstruct the mitral atrium and produce emboli. It is surgically curable. Myxedema heart disease results from a deficiency of the thyroid hormone, leading to cardiac enlargement. In some diseases there is an increase in the total output of the heart, e.g., severe anemia, hyperthyroidism, beri-beri, and where there is an arterio venous fistula.

Chapter Two

EMOTIONAL ASPECTS OF HEART DISEASE

There is a dearth of literature and even less experimental evidence on the emotional aspects of heart disease. There is more information on effect than cause. Despite the folklore—that the heart is the traditional seat of the emotions and much in literature linking the heart with courage, love, hate, etc., ("love comes from the heart," People are "soft-hearted," show "heartfelt sympathy" or are "heartless," the heart may be "bursting with joy" or "weighs on the heart," or one may die of a "broken heart,") experimental evidence of any link is hard to come by. Freud (3) called attention to the heart in connection with anxiety attacks and also in connection with various mild disorders of the heart, such as tachycardia, palpitation, and various arrhythmias, but this was purely speculation. Weiss uses the term "cardiac neurosis" where anxiety causes various abnormalities of the heart such as hypertension, various valvular defects, and what he calls "neurocirculatory asthenia." Wendkos (4) has shown alterations in the T-wave in the precordial lead in patients with neurocirculatory asthenia which cannot be distinguished from those with angina heart disease. Weiss has claimed that the pain of hypertensives and those with headaches are of the same origin. Repressed hostility (Weiss also calls it chronic rage and inhibited aggression) seems to bear a definite relationship to hypertension, and when this hostility is turned "outward," anxiety is diminished and blood pressure is often lowered. Wolf and Wolff (5) in studying patients with and without structural diseases of the heart note the following:

> "Heart pain in the presence of anatomical narrowing of the coronary arteries may result from increased work of the heart attendant upon prolonged elevation of the blood pressure and cardiac output in association with rage, resentment, anxiety, fear and tension."

They go on to say "heart pain in the presence of anatomical narrowing of the arteries may result from a fall in cardiac output and coronary blood flow in association with desperation and defeat." The latter is known as the "hypodynamic" response.

PSYCHOTHERAPY

The literature on psychotherapy with cardiacs is practically nonexistent primarily because it has been attempted so rarely. Stine (41) describes short-term psychotherapy with patients who suffered coronary insufficiency, coronary occlusion, and cardiac arrest resulting in acute anxiety and depression. Brief psychotherapy consisted of keeping the treatment goals limited to symptom relief or restoration to a previous level of functioning, early institution of treatment as soon after symptoms as possible, and focus on precipitating stress. Important elements in treatment are the early formulation of the clinical material and focusing on denial as the primary defense, attention to the narcissistic injury created by the illness or trauma, and emphasis on the cognitive understanding of the patient and of his illness.

Hickam, Cargill, and Golden (6) studied cardiovascular reaction to emotional stimuli and showed that in the majority of persons anxiety has an effect on the circulatory system similar to that produced by small doses of epinephrine.

The personality of patients with coronary artery disease has been pretty extensively studied. It might be pertinent to review these research projects.

Dunbar (7) in her monumental work in psychosomatic medicine, has delineated some of the characteristics of *her* coronary patients. There was a high illness record, a high marriage rate, they came from large families, they stuck to one job, they worked long hours without vacation under stress and strain, there was little interest in sports, there were no hobbies, and a marked interest in intellectual activities. As children they had a tendency to be stubborn and self-willed and a tendency to brood. Their early competitive relationships were with a much feared and envied parent. Their chief defense mechanisms were repression and identification. They drove themselves compulsively through hard work and self discipline but success brought no gratification or relief from tension.

Arlow (8) has made several studies on coronary patients. He describes the coronary patient as a stubborn self-willed child who very early entered into a competitive relationship with a much feared and envied parent. The conflict is repressed and an identification is made with this parent. In his work relations, there is an overwhelming drive toward success. There is also a tremendous drive toward equalling superiors and dominating others. Success does not bring with it a sense of gratification or relief from tension. The coronary individual is constantly drawn into new situations where he recreates again and again the original situation of competition. The inner insecurity and sense of weakness which these kinds of patients experience and which they deny, remains unaffected by realistic achievements. The coronary individual constantly needs new successes to alleviate his own doubts.

Miles, Waedfogel, Barrabbee and Cobb (9) studied 46 coronary patients and 49 controls in Boston. Each coronary patient and control was given a psychiatric interview of 1½ hours, a Rorschach, the 16 P F questionnaire, the Otis Mental Ability Test and their social history was reviewed. There was little discernable difference in the intensity of neurotic disturbances in the two groups, although the coronary patients tended to utilize repression to a greater degree than the controls. There was a close correlation between the character structure of the patient and his subsequent life adaptation. It was interesting that there were many more cases of cardiovascular disease reported in the families of coronary patients than in the controls; there was a two times greater incidence of histories suggesting coronary artery disease among relatives of coronary patients than in the controls, suggesting a strong familial diathesis in coronary artery disease. The coronary patients also seem less reflective than the controls. They are much more interested in action than reflection and have little awareness of their inner feelings. Coronary patients also have difficulty in handling their aggressive feelings.

Gildea (10) has summarized the views of many writers on the behavior patterns and personality factors in patients with coronary artery disease.

1. Great need for respect for authority
2. An unremitting worker
3. They stick to one occupation

4. They are invariably business executives or officials
5. They are compulsive
6. Have relatively little awareness of bodily symptoms
7. Have feelings of insecurity and inferiority
8. The work or job is a defense against anxiety
9. They are sociable and well liked.

Dr. Paul D. White, the late noted cardiologist, has made a rather plebeian but interesting note on the spiritual and physical attributes of the heart patients. He says (11) that various kinds of heart abnormalities such as cardiac enlargement, permanent arrhythmia, tachycardia, paroxymal or permanent auricular fibrillation or flutter, prolonged auricular tachycardia or heart failure may be due to emotional reasons. The most common influence of mind on the body is simple fear of heart disease. Neurocirculatory asthenia is frequently superimposed on structural heart disease. The various disorders of rhythm which may sometimes be set off by emotion may in turn cause great mental stress and on occasion have been responsible for serious neuroses.

There have been some attempts to compare the personalities of patients with various kinds of heart disease. Kemple (12) compared the personality traits of patients with rheumatic disease, hypertensive cardiovascular disease, coronary occlusion and fracture.

The rheumatics (presumably rheumatoid arthritics) show "dominant passivity and lack of aggressive drive." Many of these patients are active, energetic and even compulsively industrious. They do not identify with strong or dominant figures but with a weak dependent figure. Many of the males showed a feminine identification, a confusion about sexual roles with feelings of sexual inadequacy. In both sexes there is a prevalence of instinctive weakness and repression. Many of these patients feel acutely hostile and resentful toward various pressures in their environment and none of them find any satisfactory outlet for this hostility. Geist (13) in his extensive study of rheumatoid arthritics found that inhibited aggression is the most outstanding trait of rheumatoid arthritics.

The patients with hypertensive vascular disease, on the other hand, showed a much greater need to achieve, dominate, and be respected. They are more ambitious, more competitive. This drive to dominate appears to be an attempt to make up for inner insecurity and fear and possible weakness. They experience an acute conflict between passivity and aggressive, self assertive impulses.

The personalities of fracture patients were found to be divided into three groups—introversive, constricted, and extroverted. The first two groups showed the highest incidence of accidents. Among all the groups there is an effort to compromise between passivity and aggression with an emphasis on adaptation, self determination, independence, and day to day pleasures. The authors found that personality constriction increases with organic brain damage.

Gildea (10) compared the personality traits of people with various psychosomatic ailments. Those with the following disorders were studied: ulcerative colitis, hypertension, hyperthyroid, rheumatoid arthritis, coronary disease, peptic ulcer, and bronchial asthma. The ulcerative colitis patients were immature and narcissistic with an excessive dependence on their mothers. They gave up easily and their attacks followed stress. The hypertensives were unable to assert themselves or to express their resentment. They manifested obsessive compulsive defenses. The hyperthyroid patients had a strong attachment to their parents or parent surrogates. They were very insecure and were unable to find outlets for their emotion. They had a strong sense of responsibility. The rheumatoid arthritics were hostile and aggressive. They often found relief by abnormal, self-sacrificing helpfulness. The women tended to be tomboys, and rejecting of the feminine role. The coronary disease patients had a great need and respect for authority. They were unremitting workers and had a great deal of "sticktoitiveness." They also had obsessive compulsive defenses. The peptic ulcer patients had strong dependent needs. The onset of the ulcer was often related to life crises. Under psychotherapy they regressed to childlike dependence. The attacks of the bronchial asthma patients were related to crying. These patients were immature and had a strong need for protection. They feared separation from and are dependent on their mothers, who in many ways reject them. Very often, separation from the mother precipitated an attack. They marry late, if at all.

Hypertension has been studied by a number of investigators. Gressel et al. (14) examined 50 subjects with essential hypertension, 49 subjects without essential hypertension but with some kind of psychiatric illness, but not psychotic, and 44 subjects who had a chronic medical or surgical disorder, but not psychotic. Group I (essential hypertension) was divided into neurogenic hypertension and other types of hypertension. The "other" hypertensives were found to exhibit more obsessive compulsive behavior, and were more subnormally assertive than the other groups. The neurogenic hypertensives were shown to be not significantly different from the other kinds of hypertensives in their dynamics. The authors conclude that there is the possibility that the hypertensives are recurrently and frequently inhibiting their impulses to overt action. Franz Alexander, the renowned analyst, thinks that the compulsive traits represent an attempt to allay the anxiety which develops as a reaction to excessive hostile, destructive impulses. This corresponds closely with Gildea's findings of obsessive compulsive behavior and subnormal assertiveness in his hypertensive patients. He defined subnormal assertiveness as an inability to verbalize feelings even when aware of them. The patient simply "takes it" from boss, friends, wife, etc. These people are extremely pleasant and jovial and exhibit rare outbursts of hostility.

Rennie (15) studied four cases of essential hypertension. These patients showed lifelong instability expressed in depression and anxiety. They were also perfectionistic, ambitious and were overly attentive to bodily symptoms. These people worked at top speed, had a tremendous need to succeed and had a tendency toward jealousy and suspicion. The emotional patterns appear to be those of resentment, sometimes coupled with a desire for revenge.

The most comprehensive work on the psychological aspects of coronary artery disease has been done by Friedman and his colleagues at the Mt. Zion Hospital and Medical Center in San Francisco. The initial studies of this group began back in the 1950's. In a series of articles published in the Journal of the American Medical Association, Friedman and Rosenman studied the behavior of people with blood and cardiovascular problems. In an article in the Journal of the American Medical Association (16) three groups of men were selected solely according to their behavior pattern, which they habitually manifested in their work. The first group (Group A) of 83 were those who had an intense desire to achieve and were continually involved in competition deadlines. Eighty-three men were also chosen who had the opposite kind of behavior (Group B). The third group consisted of 46 unemployed blind men selected because they manifested a chronic state of anxiety and insecurity (Group C). Clinical coronary artery disease was seven times more frequent in group A than in group B or C. Group A men had a higher serum cholesterol, a higher frequency of arcus senilis, and a much greater smoking incidence than B, but only slightly more than C. The average ingestion of alcohol in A men was slightly higher than B, but much higher than C. The incidence of clinical artery disease in parents of A was two times that of C and one and a half times that of B. In the JAMA (17) Rosenman et al. reported on a study of 3500 men age 39-59 by various approaches to determine what characteristics of apparently well men were of predictive importance in regard to subsequent occurrence of manifest coronary heart disease. The following physiological studies were done: total serum cholesterol, blood coagulation, and cardiovascular examination. The assessment of overt behavior pattern was made by tape recorded personal interviews requiring 30 minutes. The tape recordings consisted of two monologues, one spoken by a man, the other by a woman. The male monologue was of interest to the subjects while the female's was not. The female monologue interrupted the male monologue 12 times. The total number of separating body movements and hand clenchings was recorded on the subjects listening to the male monologue. In addition, personal, parental, and socioeconomic history, smoking habits, exercise and dietary habits were assessed. Coronary patients exhibited arcus senilis eight times as frequently as normal patients and had many more frequent deformities in their respiratory and body movements.

Other findings from this study indicate that a larger number of the coronary group were in occupations having the highest level of responsibility compared with the controls. A positive history of parental coronary heart disease was obtained from 20.4% of the coronary group as compared with 17% of the controls. Although the average daily cigarette consumption by smokers did not differ significantly between the two groups, more of the coronary group were cigarette smokers. A larger number of the coronary group than controls also had a history of high blood pressure. There was no difference in blood coagulation. Higher mean beta/alpha lipoprotein levels were observed in the coronary than controls.

As a result of their studies, Friedman and Rosenman have categorized certain personality "types" as A and B. The type A man is competitive and worried that he is behind in his work, is irritable at delays in being seated on conveyances such as trains and airplanes or in being held up in traffic, is super ambitious and strives for the things held up as symbols of success in our culture—a nice house, a college education for his children, etc. This kind of person is prone to have a coronary attack.

Ginsparb and Satten (18) reviewed 20 cases of individuals who had suffered a myocardial infarction. They surmised that the coronary represents a somatic equivalent of the suicidal impulse, results from an internalization of intense aggressive impulses and that the conflict and the guilt arising from these impulses must remain totally obscured from consciousness for the conflict to be channelized into the body. They differentiate this illness from other psychosomatic illnesses which also have the symptoms of internalized aggression in that the coronary patients have a desire to "get out of this world." In a second group, the infarction seems to have developed as the individual experienced extreme rage or anger which had exceeded the physiological limits of toleration. A third group involved those individuals who seemed to be suffering what they call "emotional drain" prior to the infarct. The primary factor here is a depletion of their inner resources and inability to "give" emotionally. These are the primary personality *causes* of coronaries and infarction. The effect is depression, the mobilization of latent conflicts and needs such as the wish to be nurtured and to regress, which regression is sometimes denied resulting in the attempt at completely unattainable physical feats. In these authors' judgment, most long term survivors are found among the reality oriented individuals—wherein the patient accepts his limitations realistically and is able to reorient his life. It has been observed that these individuals are happier after the coronary than before.

Gentry, Foster and Haney (19) investigated the use of psychological tests in assessing the degree of affect manifested by patients in the intensive coronary care unit at Duke University Medical Center. Sixteen male and sixteen female patients admitted to the coronary care unit with a diagnosis of myocardial infarction were studied over a 5-day period on the unit. Half of the patients were classified as "deniers" and half as "non-deniers" based on their response to the question: "Did you feel afraid, frightened or apprehensive at any time during your hospital stay thus far?" The "deniers" answered "No" to the question while "non-deniers" responded positively. In addition, a self-report of situational anxiety and depression was obtained from each patient daily and ratings of chronic anxiety and perceived health status were obtained on days 1 and 5.

The results indicated that "deniers" reported less anxiety than "non-deniers" over the five days. The non-deniers showed a significant decrease in anxiety as time went by. Non-deniers tended to experience a marked difference between current and general health status on day 1 of the study, whereas deniers did not. The estimated level of current health was lower than that of general health on day 5, with non-deniers exhibiting marked improvement in perceived current health status to day 1. In general it was found that the defense mechanism of denial is a major determinant of the level of anxiety which characterizes these coronary patients.

Cleveland and Johnson (20) administered Rorschachs and TAT's to a group of hospitalized myocardial infarction patients and compared the results with another group of hospitalized subjects who were in a life-threatening situation and matched with the myocardial infarction patients as to age, education and socio-economic background. They found that myocardial infarction patients were more "depressive" and "agitated" than the controls. However, this was contrary to the impression that the researchers found in interviews where the myocardial infarction patients were found to be essentially achievement oriented.

Weiss et al. (21) examined young myocardial infarction patients and compared them with healthy subjects, using the clinical psychiatric interview. They concluded that the myocardial infarction patients had more psychiatric diseases and more sexual problems prior to the myocardial infarction than the controls.

Forssman and Lindegård (22) studied samples carefully matched as to somatological parameters. They found that myocardial infarction patients were more "explosive" and "hysterical" than control subjects.

Ibrahim et al. (23) compared coronary heart disease patients with "high risk" healthy subjects and with "low risk" healthy subjects ("risk" criteria were blood pressure and serum cholesterol) using the MMPI. On the basis of their results, the authors conclude that selected "coronary personality profile" (low level of manifest hostility plus elevated levels of anxiety and repression) is a result of coronary heart disease and not a cause of it.

Psychosocial factors play a considerable part in causing myocardial infarction. Various surveys in different countries have demonstrated that the incidence of myocardial infarction in young patients is related to the degree of "urbanization" of their area. The effects of treatment are the early formulation of the clinical material and focusing on denial as the primary defense, attention to the narcissistic injury created by the illness or trauma, and emphasis on the cognitive understanding of the patient of his illness. Western urbanization has been studied in Yemenite immigrants in Israel (24) and in immigrants in the U.S.A. These studies show that both serum cholesterol and myocardial incidence rise from low levels in the native countries to high levels of western urbanized areas.

Hinkle et al. (25) found that clerks without a college education had higher coronary artery incidences than clerks on the same level *with* a college education.

Kasanen et al. (26) found that those with myocardial infarction had a greater tendency not to have regular vacations, to use more soporifics and analgesics habitually and to more often consider their work hectic than did age-matched patients with other diseases. Syme et al. (27) found that people who had made four or more occupational changes had more than twice the expected prevalence of coronary heart disease. Rahe and

Paasikivi, (28) did psychosocial studies on myocardial infarction non-identical twins. In these studies the myocardial subjects proved to have experienced more excessive overtime work and more life dissatisfactions than the healthy subjects.

Van der Valk and Groen (29) found that the period prior to myocardial infarction onset was characterized by changes in many areas of the patient's life. Parkes et al. (30) discovered that the elevated mortality in men during their first months as widowers was due to myocardial infarction.

There have been a number of epidemiological studies in relation to myocardial infarction. Wardwell et al. (31) compared subjects with coronary heart disease with other controls and found that social group mobility and ethnic background were significantly discriminatory in separating the myocardial infarction group from the controls. Shekelle et al. (32) studied a group of 1500 men, ages 40-55, over a five-year period. The subjects' socio-economic and educational discrepancy from his parents and spouse were better predictors of myocardial infarction than educational and socio-economic status alone.

Theorell and his coworkers (33) have done a great deal of work in the Seraphimer Hospital, Karolinska Institutet in Stockholm, Sweden on the psychological and metabolic aspects of myocardial infarction and it might be pertinent to mention these in some detail.

Theorell devised a coronary heart disease questionnaire emphasizing work patterns, perceptions of being rushed in living patterns, and satisfaction or lack of satisfaction with several areas of life adjustment. He gave the questionnaire to 62 male subjects who had survived a myocardial infarction for a mean period of 18 months. The mean age of the group was 56 years.

The questionnaire was also given to an equal number of healthy controls. The post-myocardial infarction patients reported a higher prevalence of excessive overtime work, of dissatisfaction with their work, and greater hostility toward others when slowed down by them than the controls. The controls reported a higher prevalence of taking work home, attendance at work and non-work related organizations, supervision of others and responsibilities at work, street relaxation, physical exercise during leisure time and dissatisfaction with their financial status.

Thus the most striking observation in this phase of the study was that the patients worked overtime excessively more often than the controls. Despite the overtime, the patients lacked satisfaction in their work which they did not consider as adding to their responsibility.

Theorell gave 54 male myocardial patients with a mean age of 61.2 years a "Schedule of Recent Experience." (Twenty-seven of these patients had no previously recognized signs or symptoms of coronary heart disease while twenty-seven did have such signs during the past three years). This SRE consisted of changes in the patient's life in the past three years, such as addition of family member, in-law troubles, troubles with boss, change to a different line of work etc. (total of 36). A "life change total" was calculated and weights assigned to each life change unit (LCU) for the past 3-4 prehospitalization years. In addition, 14 friends were utilized as a control group who had no history of infarction. The infarction patients with recent episodes of coronary heart disease or other major illness showed a significant increase in LCU totals.

There have been a number of studies assessing the effect of the environment on heart disease such as temperature extremes, noise, soft water, exposure to sulfur dioxide and carbon monoxide, and constraints imposed by the community such as non-availability of high protein foods low in saturated fats and cholesterol, and limitations on physical exercise.

Various studies have shown a clear seasonal periodicity in death rates from coronary artery disease with up to 50% more deaths occurring during the winter months. Generally the increased death rate in winter occurs in those countries (and in the U.S.) where the winters are the coldest and where there is little detectable seasonal difference. A committee of the American Heart Association considered the effect of shoveling snow, for example, and concluded that this was not of major importance. In Canada, researchers have suggested that in such places as Ontario, Australia and Denmark increased heart attacks may be caused by an increase in respiratory ailments having a secondary effect on the heart. Insofar as heat is concerned, a report from Finland states that in 1970 there were 67 deaths among people taking sauna baths. On a community basis in St. Louis in 1966 there were over 300 deaths in six days during a heat wave, one-third of these attributed to atherosclerotic heart disease.

The effect of noise is uncertain and is thought to be interwoven with the whole problem of stress. Similarly, there is little evidence that exposure to ionizing radiation has increased death from heart disease (the Hiroshima survivors showed no excess of heart disease). This is particularly significant in medicine because the use of microwaves is becoming more important in medical practice.

With the problem of air pollution in the United States becoming more acute, air pollution episodes associated with high levels of sulfur dioxide (as have occurred in London and Danora) have been associated with a marked increase in deaths from atherosclerotic heart disease. However, in the main these deaths were limited to those persons with a chronic pre-existent cardio-pulmonary disease. Experimental animals that were fed cholesterol and exposed to small levels of carbon monoxide do develop atherosclerosis. It is entirely possible that this may be the reason why long-term cigarette smokers develop atherosclerosis. However, there is no conclusive proof that garage workers or people who work in enclosed tunnels show an increased risk of death from heart disease, although municipal sanitation workers in New York City, exposed to the exhaust fumes of their vehicles did have an increased death rate from coronary artery disease. It might be that driving in an automobile with closed windows in city traffic and smoking large numbers of cigarettes, may account for the coronary artery disease deaths in the larger cities.

It is thought that hard water somehow exerts a protective influence against heart disease, although the exact mechanism is not known. For example, in Monroe County, Florida (Florida Keys) the introduction of hard water from the mainland was associated with a marked drop in deaths resulting from heart disease. It may be that somehow calcium is the protective influence.

Of great importance are the prevailing living patterns within a community or group of people. On a national basis, visits to supermarkets or grocery stores show that there is little or any labeling of those items high in cholesterol or saturated fats which might be injurious to health or might precipitate cardiac difficulty. According to a recent study, the Seven Day Adventists who do not smoke, have a life expectancy in California (where the study was done) that is six years longer for males than males in the general population.

Chapter Three

ADDITIONAL CAUSES

In recent years there has been great emphasis on diet in relation to various kinds of heart disease with particular focus on the intake of saturated and unsaturated fats. While it is not the intent or function of this work to expound either on the physiological, pathological, or nutritional etiology of cardiac disease, it might be of interest to inspect some further studies in this area also done by Friedman and Rosenman. In one study (34) they obtained a detailed dietary history of 46 women and their husbands, belonging to an upper socio-economic stratum. No significant difference was found in the caloric or percentage of fat intake for each sex when corrected for difference in surface area. A critical review of various data relating to the relative immunity of the American woman to clinical coronary artery disease suggests that this immunity cannot be due entirely to some endocrine induced protection against the supposed atherogenic properties of a high fat diet. The authors conclude that probably greater stress in males causes coronary artery disease.*

The list of factors associated with the development of heart disease has grown in recent years. These include lack of physical activity, smoking, and a low concentration of certain dissolved minerals in the water supply. More recently there has been controversy about the

*It is now thought that rennin, a hormone secreted by the juxta glomerular cells of the kidney is secreted in the blood and reacts with the blood plasma to cause the formation of angiotensin which in turn produces hypertension.

etiology of heart disease due to ingestion of large amounts of coffee. In December, 1972, Jick, Slone et al. (35) observed an association between heavy coffee drinking and myocardial infarction at the Boston Collaborative Drug Surveillance Program of Boston University Medical Center. They estimated that the risk of developing myocardial infarction is about twice as great for heavy coffee drinkers as it is for those who drink no coffee at all. This conclusion was confirmed in August 1973 in a second large study by this group (36). In their first report the researchers compared 276 myocardial patients from eight hospitals in the United States, Canada, New Zealand and Israel with 1104 closely matched control pateints with other diseases. In the second study, they compared 440 white, middle-aged (age 40-69) subjects from 24 Boston area hospitals with a matched control series of 12,319 patients hospitalized with other diseases. In both studies, they found patients who drank 1-5 cups of coffee daily ran an approximately 50% greater risk of developing myocardial infarction than those who drank no coffee; patients who drank six cups daily or more ran about 110% greater risk. However, the investigators found no association between heavy coffee drinking and such closely related infarction progenitors as obesity, hypertension, and coronary insufficiency. The group also found a slight and negative correlation of coffee drinking with cigarette smoking, but there was only a slightly increased risk of infarction associated with smoking and a lesser overall risk associated with smoking than with coffee. Jick says this is consistent with previously published reports that smoking engenders the greatest risk of heart disease among individuals who are otherwise healthy, and the risk associated with smoking decreases as the risk of other factors increases.

Other investigators have obtained other results as to the relation of coffee drinking and heart disease. In the Framingham, Massachusetts Heart Disease Epidemiology Study (37), Kannell and Dawber, under the auspices of the National Institute of Health, monitored more than 5100 adult residents of Framingham over a 20-year period in an attempt to detect dietary, environmental, physiological and personality traits that increase the risk of heart disease. Their results indicate that there is no relationship between drinking coffee and heart disease.

Heyden of the Duke University Medical Center in Durham, North Carolina monitored more than 2500 results of Eruns County, Georgia for five years. He also found that there was no evidence that heart disease of any type is more frequent among those who drink large amounts of coffee (38).

Paul of the Northwestern University Medical School of Chicago monitored the health of more than 1700 middle-aged men in Chicago for three years. He reported (39) an increased incidence of heart disease among those subjects who consumed large amounts of coffee. Five years later, however, he reported that a major portion of the association between coffee and heart disease could be attributed to an association between smoking and heart disease, since heavy smokers are generally also heavy coffee drinkers and vice versa. Paradoxically he also found that the mortality rate among both smoking and non-smoking myocardial infarction victims was lower for coffee drinkers than for non-drinkers and that smokers who are heavy coffee drinkers run less risk of developing myocardial infarctions than smokers who are non-drinkers.

There have been a number of smaller studies which have produced contradictory results. For example,

Wilhelmin and Tribben (40) in Sweden have monitored the health of 835 residents of Gothenburg since 1963 (10 years). They found no association between coffee drinking and heart disease. Thiel and his associates at the University of Oklahoma School of Medicine compared 50 subjects with an equal number of closely matched controls and found a significantly increased consumption of fluids including coffee among myocardial infarction patients. Other small scale studies have generally revealed no link between coffee consumption and heart disease, although nearly all investigators have noted strong correlations between coffee drinking and smoking, and between smoking and heart disease.

In addition to diet, other risk factors have been studied. An interesting continuing study being conducted by Wilmore at the University of California Medical Center in San Francisco, California investigated whether the effect of the risk factor can be cancelled by a change in the person's life style such as a carefully programmed exercise regimen. The interesting element of this study is that the subjects are 95 schoolboys ranging in age from 8-12 years, who come from two public schools in Davis, California. They are healthy, well-fed, relatively affluent and far above average compared with the national norms for endurance and stamina. In addition to being weighed regularly, measurements are taken of body fat, cholesterol, and EKG's. They are also given a battery of endurance tests. Of the 95, 36 were on the borderline of obesity while 12 were obese; there was a significantly high cholesterol level in eight youngsters; 32 had a family history of heart attack under age 60; and abnormal EKG's were taken at rest for two boys and after exercise in three. The boys from one of the Davis schools have been given a special exercise program while the boys from the other program have continued with their normal school physical education activities. The results of this study have not yet been published.

Chapter Four

PATIENTS, QUESTIONNAIRE AND RESULTS

The Patients

The patients in this project were both hospitalized and ambulatory, and all were afflicted with cardiac disease in the following categories:

I. Arteriosclerotic Heart Disease—patients with angina pectoris, acute myocardial infarction and coronary artery disease.

II. Hypertensive Vascular Disease—patients with essential hypertension, renal hypertension, malignant hypertension and endocrine disturbances.

III. Disturbances of Conduction—patients with S. A. or A. V. block.

IV. Valvular Disease—patients with mitral stenosis, mitral insufficiency, aortic insufficiency, tricuspid stenosis and tricuspid insufficiency.

Diagnosis was made by the cardiologist in the hospital or clinic or if a private patient, by the patient's personal physician. See Table I for a summary of the patients and their diagnosis.

Table No 1

DIAGNOSES

N-124

ARTERIOSCLEROTIC HEART DISEASE*	
ASHD (%)	66
Myocardial infarction	26
Myocardial insufficiency(%)	03
Angina (%)	10

N-87

HYPERTENSIVE CARDIOVASCULAR DISEASE	
Hypertension (%)	100

N-72

VALVULAR*	
Aortic insufficiency (%)	57
Rheumatic heart disease (%)	22
Valve replacement (%)	14
Mitral Stenosis (%)	07
Subacute bacterial endocarditis (%)	07

N-56

DISTURBANCE OF CONDUCTION*	
Heart block or complete heart block (%)	50
Congestive heart failure (%)	33
Bilateral bundle branch block(%)	17
Disturbance of conduction (%)	17

* The total is more than 100% since some patients had more than one diagnosis.

QUESTIONNAIRE[1]

The questionnaire was designed to assess various psychological aspects of the patient's disease, but other areas also were explored. In addition to identifying data such as age, sex, diagnosis, medication, marital status, data symptoms first noticed and what they were, the life change unit (LCU) self concept was explored. Such information as kinds of psychological disturbance at time of occurrence of symptoms, i.e., stress, loss of someone close before or after symptoms, difficulty with career or money, were assessed. Various other psychosomatic manifestations such as headache, enuresis, tics, were also assessed both during childhood and adulthood. Subjective estimates of psychological variables such as ambition, persistence, dependency, expression of grief and rage, conformity were obtained. Frequency and type of nocturnal dreams and day-dreams were also assessed. Familial information such as personality of parents, which parent was dominant in the home, family attitude toward heart disease, incidence of psychosomatic ailments in family were collated. A fairly detailed work history on each patient was obtained including how well the patient got along with employees, employers and other superiors. Strength of religious belief was obtained for each patient. Elements tangential to psychological variables were obtained from each patient such as alcohol ingestion, smoking, use of drugs, diet, and exercise previous to and after symptoms were assessed.[2] Finally, satisfaction with current treatment was asked of each patient.

[1]see appendix for full questionnaire.

[2]At the time the heart patients were being questioned, coffee drinking was not thought to have any influence on the etiology of heart disease.

ANALYSIS OF QUESTIONNAIRE

The questionnaire was analyzed for information both *within* each cardiac group and *between* cardiac groups. Inasmuch as numbers are meaningless, the *percentages* in each category of heart disease were computed.

ARTERIOSCLEROTIC HEART DISEASE

Here the number of subjects was slightly in favor of males—59% males to 41% females. The average age of each sex was almost exactly the same—58.65 years for males and 58.92 years for females. Interestingly, the largest percentage was widowed and the next largest were married. Forty five percent had some relatives with heart disease, indicating that to some extent this type of heart disease has a familial diathesis. Of this group with someone in the family having heart disease, in the largest number (18%) the father was afflicted, with the next largest the mother (15%). Eight-five percent of this group had their heart disease for over two years and only 15% had the disease under 2 years. Only a small fraction of those with this kind of heart disease (17%) had lost someone close to them at the time of the appearance of symptoms, and only 10% of this group said they had financial problems at the time of the appearance of symptoms. The conception of how disabled they were due to this type of heart disease ranged from moderately (52%) to severely disabled (45%) with only 3% stating that they were not disabled at all. A total of 97% of this group thought they were either moderately or totally disabled. As one might expect, the reaction of relatives to the patient's illness was greatest—38% of the relatives greatly upset by the appearance of the disease as against 24% of friends and 16% of acquaintances being greatly upset. In both acquaintances and friends the largest group was moderately upset and a goodly percentage of the relatives moderately upset. Another interesting finding in this type of heart disease is that a goodly number, 84%, had lost some close relatives by death just previous to the symptoms, spread rather evenly by husband (16%), wife (14%), father (14%), brother (14%), and mother (10%). This suggests that loss of a close relative may precipitate an attack of this type of heart disease. Insofar as other psychosomatic ailments having hysterical components are concerned, either as a child or adult, headaches, temper tantrums, tremors, and heart pains do seem to have some relationship to this kind of heart disease—35% had headaches as a child (16% one per week and 19% one per month); 30% had headaches as an adult (15% very often—one per day and 15% one every three days) and 38% one per month. Only a small percentage had tremors as a child but 27% had tremors either one per week or one per month as an adult (15% one per week and 12% one per month). Twenty-seven percent had temper tantrums either one per week or one per month as a child (12% one per week and 15% one per month) while 20% admitted to temper tantrums once every three days, one per week or one per month (4% once every three days, 4% once every week and 12% once a month). Sixteen percent said they had cardiac pain as a child either once a week or once a month (4% once a week and 12% once a month), while as might be expected, 69% said they currently had heart pains once a month or more (15% every day; 15% one every three days; 27% one every week and 12% once a month). Practically none of these patients admitted to having tics, convulsions, enuresis, or to having stuttered, bitten their nails or sucked their thumb either as a child or adult. Only a small fraction of these patients got angry easily (18%)[1]. A goodly percentage (38%) said they withdrew from difficult situations, but the majority said they did not. It is rather interesting that most of these patients had a high regard for themselves insofar as certain psychological traits are concerned. Eighty-seven percent said they were ambitious, 79% said they were persistent, 100% said they were in good control of themselves, 100% said they were clean, 85% said they were independent, and 74% said they were *not* moody. Insofar as *expression* of certain emotions is concerned, approximately half were able to express joy and grief; 92% were able to express rage[2] and 86% other emotions. As might be expected, since this is an older group, 100% did conform to current mores.

Analysis of Dreams

All of these patients dreamed at night, with 8% dreaming practically every night, 36% once every few nights, and 28% one night per week; 28% dreamed less than one night per week. Fifty eight percent had very clear dreams, 25% moderately clear, and 17% had jumbled up dreams. Four percent dreamed all night, 17% half the night, and 79% less than half the night. Forty six percent had daytime fantasies and 54% did not. Of the group that did have daydreams, 18% had them every day, and 27% once every few days. One hundred percent saw these daydreams as either very (56%) or moderately (44%) clear, while none saw them as jumbled up. Evidently such pleasantries as vacation (20%)

[1]Contrast this with the results on rheumatoid arthritis patients. See Geist, H. *The Psychological Aspects of Rheumatoid Arthritis,* C.C. Thomas and Co., 1966 pp. 39-40.

[2]Ibid. p. 42

or money (20%) constituted 40% of the subject matter of this group's dreams while 13% dreamed of things related to work.

Eighty two percent of this group got along either very well with their mother (17%) or well (65%) while 18% got along fairly well or poorly. Sixty eight percent got along with the father either very well (5%) or well (63%) while 32% got along fairly well or poorly. [*None* of this group got along *very* well with their siblings but 67% got along well and 24% got along fairly well, or poorly (9%).] It is rather interesting that in most of this group the mother was the disciplinarian in the family (64%) with the father the disciplinarian only 32%.

In 62% of the cases here, the family either accepted or were indifferent to the disease and in only 14% of the cases was the family upset. However 14% said that the affliction was a serious problem to the family.

Only 31% of the arteriosclerotic group had either psychosomatic ailments in the family or had other psychosomatic ailments themselves. *None* of the fathers had these while 33% of the mothers and 67% of some other member of the family had these diseases.

The average time spent on the job was 10.94 years with a range from 2 months to 43 years. Eighty eight percent of the respondents said they enjoyed their job and all said they got along with the boss and other people on the job. Ninety two percent said they got along with their previous bosses while 100% said the got along with previous co-workers.

The majority of these patients are moderately religious (44%), i.e., go to a place of worship occasionally and observe some holidays while 19% said they were extremely religious, i.e., worship regularly and observe all religious holidays. Thirty seven percent rarely (26%) or never (11%) go to any place of worship.

Since the intake of drugs, alcohol, diet, and exercise are crucial to this study, a statistical tabulation of these variables will be made last.

A large majority (70%) said they felt good about the doctor examining them or it didn't bother them.* Thirty seven percent said their symptoms increased when they were emotionally upset, while 63% said they did not. Sixty five percent said their symptoms increased when they exercised, while 35% said they did not. Forty six percent said their symptoms increased earlier under adverse weather conditions. Of this group, 41% said they increased in humid or rainy weather, while 35% in cold weather and 24% in hot weather. Allied with this, 42% said their symptoms increased at certain seasons of the year. Of this group, 70% said their symptoms increased during the winter months, while 30% said they increased during the summer months.

RECAPITULATION OF ARTERIOSCLEROTIC HEART DISEASE GROUP

The arteriosclerotic heart disease patients were essentially a middle aged, mostly widowed, "establishment" group. These patients also had a familial cardiac diathesis, mostly on the mother's side but none on the father's. Temper tantrums and tremors seemed to be two of the symptomatologies associated with hysterical psychosomatic psychopathology both as a child and adult. Although they thought themselves either moderately or severely disabled because of their ailment, they had an unusually high regard for themselves and

*The majority of the ASHD patients were clinic patients but some were hospitalized or ambulatory patients of private physicians.

good self concept. In the growing and formative years, they got along well with all members of the family, with the mother rather than the father being the disciplinarian. Their work history was good, having worked for an average of 10 years on the job and according to their subjective reports got along with bosses and colleagues. They were a combination of moderately or extremely religious. The two elements which exacerbated their symptoms were exercise and adverse weather conditions.

HYPERTENSIVE VASCULAR DISEASE

In this group, 40% were males and 60% females. The average age was about the same, 55 years for males and 53.7 years for females. The greater majority of these patients were single (40%), while 20% were divorced, 20% widowed, and 20% separated. None of these patients had anyone in the family with heart disease. All had their disease over 2 years. Twenty percent had lost someone close to them just previous to symptoms. All of this group thought they were seriously (40%) or moderately (60%) disabled because of their heart disease. Seventy five percent of the relatives of this group were moderately upset, while 25% were indifferent to the patients with this kind of disease. Of these patients' friends, 100% were moderately upset, while 75% of their acquaintances were mildly upset, and 25% indifferent. Fifty percent of these patients had lost a mother just before symptoms; 16% had lost a child or husband.

As children, all of these patients had headaches either quite often (40% once every 3 days) or moderately often (60% between once a week and once a month), 20% had headaches every day, and 80% once a month or less, as an adult. Twenty percent had tremors everyday as a child, and 80% once a month or less as a child; 40% had tremors every day as an adult, while 60% had tremors between once a week and once a month. None of these patients had tics, convulsions, stuttered, bit nails or sucked his thumb, or had enuresis either as a child or adult. Significantly, however, 40% had temper tantrums as a child every day, while 60% had temper tantrums as a child between once a week and once a month. Twenty percent had temper tantrums as an adult every day. Twenty percent had heart pains every day as a child; 40% had heart pains once every 3 days; 60% had heart pains between once a week and once a month as an adult. In this group of heart patients, 60% said they got angry easily, and 40% did not; 60% withdrew from difficult situations while 40% did not. All of these patients thought they were ambitious, persistent, in good control of themselves, and clean, while 80% thought they were moody, independent, and adequate. All of them were able to express joy and other emotions (other than joy, grief and rage); 60% were able to express grief and grief and rage); 60% were able to express grief and There were no renegades in this group. All said they conformed to everyday mores. Insofar as dreams were concerned, all of them dreamed, with 80% dreaming either once every few nights or one night per week, while the remainder dreamed practically every night. Eighty percent had very clear dreams while the remainder had dreams which were moderately clear. All of this group dreamed less than half the night. Sixty percent daydreamed, while 40% did not. Of this 60%, all of them daydreamed once every few days and all had daydreams which were moderately clear. The content of the dreams were divided equally between illness, future, money, clothes, food, travel, and excitement. All of this group got along well with the mother, father and siblings. In half of the group the mother was the disciplinarian and in the other half, the father. Fifty percent of this group didn't know how their family reacted to the heart disease, while only 25% said their family was sympathetic. Twenty percent of these hypertensive patients had family members with psychosomatic ailments.

The average length on the job was 14.25 years with a range of 7-30 years. All of this group said they enjoyed their work, got along with their boss in their immediate and past work.

Seventy five percent of this group were either extremely (25%) or moderately (50%) religious while 25% rarely went to any place of worship.

Sixty percent of this group felt good about the doctor examining them while 20% said it didn't bother them, and 20% said they resisted it. All of them were satisfied with the treatment they were getting.

Eighty percent of these patients said their symptoms increased when they were emotionally upset and of this group, 20% claimed anxiety, 20% depression, 60% "pressured"—which increased their symptoms. Forty percent said that exercise increased their symptoms, 40% said certain weather conditions made their symptoms worse (half rain and half heat), while 40% said their symptoms were worse during certain seasons (divided equally among Fall, Spring, and Summer), and none said their symptoms were increased at other times.

These patients were of a single, middle aged, "established" religious group where heart disease in the family seemed to be no factor, although a large number had lost their mother (not by heart disease) just previous to symptoms. They perceived themselves as either moderately or severely disabled because of their heart disease. Headaches were predominant as an hysterical psychosomatic symptom both as a child and adult, with tremors also present to some extent as a child. Temper tantrums were also present as a child. A large majority of these patients got angry easily and also withdrew from difficult situations. In general, they had good self concept and got along with all members of the family while growing up. They had an excellent work record, with an average of 14 years on the job, and according to their own assertions got along with their bosses and colleagues. Emotional upset brought about an exacerbation of symptoms.

VALVULAR DISEASE

There were 57% males and 43% females in this group. The average age of the males was 43.13 years and the average age of the females 40.5 years. Most of these patients were separated (36%), while 29% were married, 14% divorced, 14% single, and 7% widowed. Half of these patients had someone else in the family with heart disease: mother—22%; brother—11%; father—6%; sister—6%; wife—6%. Seventy one percent had their ailment over 2 years, and 29% under 2 years. Twenty one percent had difficulty with money just previous to their heart disease. Another 21% had lost someone close to them just previous to their heart disease. Seventy one percent thought they were moderately disabled due to their heart disease, 14% thought they were severely disabled, and 15% not at all disabled. Forty six percent of the relatives were moderately upset about the patient's heart problem, 23% were indifferent, 23% greatly upset, and 8% were mildly upset. Approximately the same figures were true of friends: 43% were moderately upset, 21% indifferent, 21% greatly upset, 7% mildly upset, and 7% had other reactions. Twenty seven percent of the acquaintances were either greatly or moderately upset, 18% indifferent, and 9% other reactions. Twenty nine percent of these patients lost their mother just previous to symptoms, while 17% lost a husband, 11% a wife, and 6% a father, sister or aunt. Twenty four percent had not lost anyone just prior their symptoms.

Headaches and temper tantrums were the only two psychosomatic variables with any "significant" incidence in this group either as a child or adult. Twenty one percent had headaches: quite often (14%) moderately often (7%); while 21% had headaches hardly ever as a child. The occurrence of headaches as an adult was somewhat greater, with 21% having them quite often and 14% moderately often. Twenty one percent had temper tantrums as a child: quite often (7%); moderately often (14%). But as an adult none had temper tantrums either very often or quite often, and only 7% had temper tantrums moderately often. In all the other variables, the incidence was negligible, although again as might be expected, 14% had heart pains quite often, and 43% had heart pains moderately often as an adult. Thirty one percent of this group said they got angry easily, and 43% said they withdrew from difficult situations. A large majority of these patients said they were ambitious (71%), persistent (92%), in good control of themselves (93%), moody (71%), clean (100%), independent (69%), and adequate (86%). As for expressions of emotions, 54% were *unable* to express grief, all were able to express joy, 75% able to express rage, and all able to express other emotions. Seventy seven percent were able to conform to everyday mores. All of these patients dreamed at one time or another, with 8% dreaming practically every night, 25% once every few nights, and 8% one night per week; 59% dreamed less than one night per week; Eighty four percent had dreams which were either very clear (42%) or moderately clear (42%). Most (78%) of these patients dreamed less than half the night. Thirty nine percent of this group had daydreams, with 80% daydreaming either practically every day (20%) or once every few days (60%). Half had very clear daydreams and half moderately clear. A large number (25%) daydreamed about money, with 13% daydreaming about vacations or work, and 49% about other things. Ninety two percent of these patients got along well (85%) or very well (7%) with their mother. Seventy percent got along very well (10%) or well (60%) with their father. None got along very well with their siblings but 77% got along well. In most of the families of these patients (65%), the father was the disciplinarian, while in the remainder the mother was the disciplinarian (35%). Fifty percent of the families of this group saw the patient's heart disease either as a serious problem or were sympathetic (25%), 17% were indifferent, 8% accepted the situation, and 25% didn't know how their families felt about the heart disease. Thirty three percent of these patients had someone in the family with some kind of psychosomatic ailment, and of this group none was the mother or father; all the ailments occurred in some other relatives. Average stay on the job was 4.77 years ranging from 2 months to 11 years. Seventy three percent said they enjoyed their work and all said they got along with their boss and colleagues in their job just previous to their heart attack and previous jobs.

Insofar as religion was concerned, this group had about an equal spread among all categories: 31% were extremely religious, 23% moderately religious, 23% went to place of worship sometimes, and 23% never.

Seventy seven percent said they felt good about the doctor examining them, while 23% said it didn't bother them. All were satisfied with the treatment they were getting. Fifty four percent said that their symptoms increased when they got emotionally upset, and 54% said that their symptoms increased when they exercised. Only 15% said that their symptoms increased under certain weather conditions (50% hot weather, 50% cold weather), and 31% during certain seasons (75% summer, 25% winter).

RECAPITULATION OF VALVULAR GROUP

These patients were also a middle aged "establishment" group but considerably younger than the arteriosclerotic or hypertensive groups. Their heart disease was chronic (over two years). They thought their disease was either moderately or severely disabling. The majority of relatives or friends were moderately or greatly upset due to their heart disease. A large number lost their mother just previous to the appearance of symptoms. Headaches and temper tantrums were two hysterical psychosomatic symptoms which were present in these patients both as a child and adult. All of them reported a good self concept. All seemed to get along with their mother and father in their formative years, and in this group the father was the disciplinarian. Their work history was fairly good but not as good as the arteriosclerotics and hypertensives. All claimed to have gotten along well with colleagues and bosses on the job. A majority said their symptoms increased when they were emotionally upset.

DISTURBANCE OF CONDUCTION

In this group, 67% were males and 33% females. The average age of the males was 60 years; females 62.5 years. Fifty percent of these patients were single, while 17% were divorced, 17% married, and 16% separated, while none were widowed. Forty three percent of these patients had someone in the family with heart disease, equally divided among father, brother, grandfather, and son. Eighty percent had their affliction over 2 years, and 20% under 2 years. Seventeen percent had lost someone close to them just before their symptoms, while 34% had money problems just previous to their symptoms. Fifty percent of these patients thought they were moderately disabled, while 33% thought they were severely disabled, and 17% not at all disabled (83% moderately or severely disabled). Of their relatives, friends, and acquaintances, 67% of the relatives were moderately upset by the patients' heart ailment, while 33% were greatly upset; 80% of the friends were moderately upset, while 20% of the friends were greatly upset; the same figures were true of acquaintances. Of those who had lost someone close just before symptoms, they were divided equally (17% among father, mother, husband, and son). Of the psychosomatic ailments assessed, symptomatology as a child was noticeably absent, except for temper tantrums and heart pains. However, a large number of these patients did have symptomatology of headaches, tremors, and surprisingly enough enuresis, temper tantrums, and heart pains. Sixty seven percent of these patients had temper tantrums moderately often as a child, while 17% had heart pains very often as a child. However, 20% had headaches quite often, or moderately often (40%) as an adult; 17% had tremors either very often or moderately often 17%). Seventeen percent were enuretic moderately often as an adult while 33% had temper tantrums moderately often as an adult. Seventeen percent currently had heart pains moderately often, 33% of these patients got angry easily, while half withdrew from difficult situations and half did not. All claimed to be ambitious and persistent, while 84% said they were in good control of themselves. Half said they were moody, while half said they were not. All thought they were clean. Sixty seven percent said that they were independent and all thought they were adequate. Sixty seven percent said that they were able to express grief, 83% able to express joy, 33% able to express rage, and 60% able to express other emotions. All said they comformed to everyday mores.

All of these patients said they dreamed, with 33% dreaming practically every night, 33% once every few nights, and 17% one night every few weeks. Eighty four percent of these patients' dreams were either very clear or moderately clear. Most of them dreamed less than half the night (67%); 33% daydreamed, while 67% did not. Of the 33%, half daydreamed practically every day, while half daydreamed less than one day per week. All of them had very clear daydreams. Of those that did daydream, half daydreamed about accomplishments, and half about discipline. Eighty percent of these patients got along very well (20%), or well (60%) with their mother while 75% got along well with their father, and 25% only fair. Fifty percent got along well with their sibs; 25% fair; and 25% poorly. In 50% of the cases, the mother was the disciplinarian; 33% the father; 17% somebody else. In 33% of the group, the patients didn't know how their family felt about their heart disease; 33% were in some other category than that assessed by the questionnaire. In 17% the family was indifferent, and in 17% the family thought it was a serious problem. Thirty three percent had someone in the family with psychosomatic ailments, with 33% the mother, and 67% some other members of the family. The average length on the job of this group was 2 years. Considering that the average age for males was 60 years and 62.5 years for females, this was really short duration of job tenure.

Fewer of these patients (80%) said they got along with their boss well than the other types of heart patients. The same holds true as to enjoying their job (80%) and getting along with others on the job (75%). The percentage are even lower for past work with 50% getting along well with their boss and 50% either fair or badly; 50% got along well with others in their past work and 50% fairly well.

The majority of these patients were moderately religious (60%), while 40% said they rarely went to a place of worship.

Fifty percent said that they feel good about the doctor examining them, while 50% said it dosen't bother them. All were satisfied with the treatment they were getting. Eighty three percent said that their symptoms were increased when they were emotionally upset, half said their symptoms increased when they exercised, one-third said their symptoms increased under certain weather conditions (cold 33%, damp 33%, and heat 34%). One-third said their symptoms increase during a certain season (⅓ Spring, ⅓ Winter, and ⅓ Summer). One-third said their symptoms increased at other times (50% when tired, and 50% when they argued with their children).

RECAPITULATION OF DISTURBANCE OF CONDUCTION

This group of patients had the highest average age of all the patients. However, they were also an "establishment" group, most of whom were single. Their affliction was chronic and there seems to be a familial diathesis in their disease. The majority thought they were either seriously or moderately disabled. Relatives, friends, and acquaintances were quite upset by their heart ailment. Thus, it appears that this kind of cardiac disease (disturbance of conduction) does upset those surrounding the patient. Headaches, tremors, and temper tantrums were currently present and a goodly number had temper tantrums as a child. Insofar as self concept is concerned, the positive self concept expressed by other cardiac patients was not as unanimous in this group. The chief difference in the variables was in moodiness where half said they were moody and 37% said they were dependent. Their job tenure was relatively short. Of all the cardiac patients, this group got along less well with their bosses and colleagues than the others. A goodly number said their symptoms increased under emotional stress.

Since this was an older set of patients, all groups were "establishment" and conformed to current mores. Their heart affliction was chronic. The oldest group included those who suffered from disturbance of conduction, and in descending chronological order: arteriosclerotic heart disease, hypertensive vascular disease, and valvular disease. The marital state of these patients is an interesting phenomenon, being widely divergent. The hypertensive and disturbances of conduction groups were primarily single, the arteriosclerotic primarily widowed, and the valvular separated. Just why this is so is not clear, since it might be postulated that the stresses of married life might precipitate almost any kind of heart disease, yet in none of these groups was the married state predominant. It may be that the precipitants are independent of the marital state. The arteriosclerotic group had a definite familial diathesis, while the valvular and disturbance of conduction groups have a possible familial diathesis. Loss of someone, particularly the mother, just previous to symptoms was characteristic of the arteriosclerotic hypertensive, and valvular but not the disturbance of conduction group. Temper tantrums and tremor are a surprising set of syndromes both as a child and adult in the arteriosclerotic heart patients, and headaches in the hypertensive patients, while headaches and temper tantrums were evidenced in the valvular group; headache, tremor and temper tantrums were present in the disturbance of conduction group. Practically all of the heart patients in each group thought themselves moderately disabled. In each group, except for disturbance of conduction, the patients had a universally high regard for themselves according to their self reports. All got along well with members of their family while they were growing up. Disciplinarian in the family varied with the mother in the arteriosclerotic, father in hypertensives and split evenly between mother and father in the other two groups. In none of these patients were psychosomatic ailments present to any extent in relatives. The hypertensives were the only group that got angry easily and withdrew from difficult situations. All patients, according to their subjective reports, had a good work history (previous to heart condition) getting along with bosses and colleagues. Length on the job varied from a mean of 2 years in the disturbance of conduction group, to 14 years in the hypertensive group. Emotional upset caused an exacerbation of symptoms with a majority of all patients except the arteriosclerotic.

ALCOHOL, SMOKING, DRUGS, EXERCISE AND FATTY FOODS

Because of the controversy about and importance of these elements in relation to heart disease, they will be considered separately in each category of heart disease, and also as a whole.

Arteriosclerotic Heart Disease

In this group, 19% imbibed alcohol either more than once a week or once a week (22%) previous to this heart condition, while 44% imbibed alcohol less than once per week, with 15% never touching alcohol. In relation to the general population and the incidence of inebriation, this is a considerable number of people with arteriosclerotic heart disease who imbibed alcohol either often or very often. Thirty three percent smoked more than one pack of cigarettes a day, while 44%

smoked less than one pack a day, and 22% did not smoke. None of these heart patients smoked about a pack a day. Sixty nine percent of these heart patients took only their medication and no other drugs, 14% took anacin in additon to their medication, while 17% took other drugs. Of this 17% who took other drugs, all took them orally with half taking them every day and half about one day per month. Fifty six percent had exercised either a great deal or moderately just previous to their heart attack while 44% exercised mildly, with none never exercising. Fifty three percent ate fatty foods either in large (15%) or moderate amounts (38%); 29% ate fatty foods in small amounts, while only 18% never ate fatty foods.

Hypertensive Vascular Disease

In the hypertensive vascular disease group, none imbibed alcohol more than once per week—25% once per week, and the remaining 75% took alcohol less than once per week. None of these patients smoked more than one pack per day—25% smoked about one pack per day and the remaining 75% smoked less than a pack per day. None of these patients did not smoke at all. Sixty seven percent took no drugs exclusive of medication, while 17% took only aspirin, and 16% took other pills (unspecified). All of these patients took the "other" drugs orally. Of these patients, 25% exercised a great deal, or moderately (75%) previous to their heart attack, while none did not exercise at all. Twenty five percent ate fatty foods a great deal previous to their heart attack, none ate fatty foods moderately, 25% ate small amounts of fatty foods, and 50% never ate fatty foods.

Valvular Disease

In the valvular disease group, 8% imbibed alcohol

more than once a week, or once a week (46%), 38% rarely touched alcohol, and 8% were teetotalers. Twenty three percent either smoked more than one pack per day, or one pack per day (39%), 15% smoked less than a pack a day, while 23% did not smoke at all. Twenty three percent exercised either a great deal or moderately, while 23% exercised mildly, and 8% not at all. Fifty eight percent of this group took no drugs other than their medication, while 17% took aspirin. Eight percent took "illegal" drugs (grass, speed, etc.), 8% took qualude, and 8% took other drugs. All who took "other" drugs took them orally. Twenty three percent exercised a great deal, or moderately (46%), 23% mildly and only 8% never exercised previous to their heart disorder. Twenty three percent ate fatty foods a great deal, or moderately (46%) previous to their cardiac affliction, 31% ate small amounts of fatty foods, and none *never* ate fatty foods.

Disturbances of Conduction

In the disturbance of conduction group, 20% imbibed alcohol moderately, and 80% rarely. Twenty percent smoked more than one pack per day, none about a pack a day, none less than a pack a day, and 80% did not smoke or never smoked. None of these patients took any drugs other than their medication. Twenty percent of these patients ate fatty foods a great deal, 20% moderately and the remainder in small amounts.

Results for all groups

In the cardiac group as a whole, 12% imbibed alcohol a great deal or moderately (29%), while 45% imbibed rarely and 14% not at all. Twenty seven percent smoked more than one pack a day, or about a pack a day (9%), 31% less than a pack a day, and 33% never smoked. Sixteen percent exercised a great deal, or moderately (38%), 41% mildly, and 4% not at all previous to their heart attack. Eighteen percent ate fatty foods either a great deal, or moderately (35%), 31% small amounts, and 14% never ate fatty foods.

RECAPITULATION OF INFLUENCES IN VARIOUS KINDS OF HEART DISEASE

In all the different kinds of heart disease, ingestion of fatty foods seem to be a significant eating pattern in patients just previous to their heart disease. Ingestion in either moderate or large amounts of alcohol previous to their heart attack seems to be a factor in *arteriosclerotic heart disease* and *valvular disease,* but not in the other. In only those patients with valvular disease does smoking appear to be a factor. Since practically all of these patients exercised a good deal previous to their heart attack, it could not be ascertained whether lack of exercise might have an influence on the etiology of any specific kind of heart disease. Drugs taken previous to the affliction seems to have no influence whatsoever.

Chapter Five

THE STATISTICAL DESIGN
BC TRY SYSTEM

A cluster analysis is a method of objectively grouping together entities on the basis of their similarities or differences. When the entities compared are variables such as mental abilities or personality traits, the procedure is called "cluster analysis of variables" or simply "V analysis". It was previously labelled "factor analysis", a term still used, though strictly speaking it refers only to the mathematical procedures of analyses called "factoring". The term cluster analysis applies equally well to entities that are objects such as persons. The procedure of grouping together objects that have similar patterns or characteristics is known as cluster analysis of objects or simply "O analysis". This cluster analysis is one of the procedures used in nearly all fields of human thought and scientific study. The specific program in this cluster analysis is the BC TRY SYSTEM of cluster and factor analysis. The BC TRY SYSTEM was developed by the late Professor Robert Tryon, Professor of Psychology at the University of California in Berkeley. It includes programs such as cluster analyses on as many as 2,000 variables (known as the BIGN analysis). In a cluster analysis, the procedure consists essentially of an input mechanism, control data cards, the system tape containing the programs which perform the factor or cluster analysis and the executive program putting these components into operation, and data storage tape used for further analysis. The monitor output tapes contain all printed and punched output available to the user.

In the BC TRY SYSTEM as applied to this project, the variables which clustered together to form 3 factors were delineated. Then those heart disease patients which clustered on these factors were ascertained. Finally the *groups* of cardiac patients which clustered on each factor were also ascertained. In this way I could ascertain the personality variables for each group of cardiac patients.

The variables in the BC TRY program were essentially scales of various personality tests.* These were as follows:

Test I—Multiple Affect Check List—Today Form

This instrument was chosen because it is relatively short and is not taxing on the energy and resources of the subject. Since heart patients were being tested, the author did not think it feasible to use instruments like the MMPI which might tax the resources of these patients. The test consists of 132 adjectives measuring "affect traits" in which the examinee is asked to check those adjectives describing how he feels the day he takes the test and also how he feels in general. The best definition of the scales is embodied in some of the items in them.

Variable # I

A. Anxiety—	[x*]afraid	desperate	[x]fearful
[x]frightened	[x]nervous	[x]panicky	[x]shaky
[x]tense	terrified	[x]upset	[x]worrying

Variable # 2

B. Depression—

destroyed	[x]discouraged	[x]forlorn	[x]gloomy
[x]hopeless	[x]lonely	[x]lost	[x]low
[x]miserable	[x]rejected	sad	[x]suffering
[x]sunk	[x]terrible	[x]tormented	[x]wilted

*The reader can obtain information concerning the tests used in this study from the psychological literature.

Variable # 3

C. Hostility—	^{x}angry	bitter	^{x}cruel
^{x}disagreeable	discontented	disgusted	enraged
furious	irritated	^{x}mad	mean
offended	outraged	stormy	unsociable
vexed			

*X refers to items showing high correlation with full test.

Variable # 4

Test II—Cardiac Adjustment Scale

This is a test of 160 items which determines readiness of cardiacs for safe return to work.

Test III—Tennessee Self Concept Scale (Counseling Form)

This is an instrument which measures self concept. The individual's concept of himself has been demonstrated to be highly influential in determining his behavior and is also related to his general personality and state of mental health. The total scale consists of 100 self descriptive statements which the subject uses to portray his own picture of himself. Various scores or areas of self concept are delineated. Those used in this study are as follows:

Variable # 5

1. Self Criticism Score (SC): High scores indicates a normal openness and capacity for self criticism.

Variable # 6

2. Total P Score: Persons with high scores tend to like themselves, feel they are persons of value and worth and have confidence in themselves.

Variable # 7

3. Row 1 P Score—Identity: These are "what I am"

items. Here the individual is describing his basic identity—what he is as he sees himself.

Variable # 8

4. Row 2 P Score—Self Satisfaction: This score reflects the level of self satisfaction or self acceptance. High scores indicate great self satisfaction and great self acceptance.

Variable # 9

5. Row 3 P Score—Behavior: This score measures the individual's perception of his own behavior in the way he functions.

Variable # 10

6. Column A—Physical Self: Here the individual is presenting his view of his body, his state of health, his physical appearance, skills and sexuality. High scores indicate positive attitudes toward these areas.

Variable # 11

7. Column B—Moral Ethical Self: This score describes the self from a moral-ethical frame of reference—moral worth, relationship to God, feelings of being a "good" or "bad" person and satisfaction with one's religion or lack of it. High scores indicate perception of self as positive in the moral-ethical area.

Variable # 12

8. Column C—Personal Self: This score reflects the individual's sense of personal worth, his feeling of adequacy as a person and his evaluation of his personality apart from his body or relationship to others. High scores indicate a good sense of personal worth.

Variable # 13

9. Column D—Family Self: This score reflects one's feeling of adequacy, worth and value as a family member. High scores indicate perception of self as a good family member.

Variable # 14

10. Column E—Social Self: This reflects the person's sense of adequacy and worth in his social interaction with other people in general. High scores indicate high sense of worth in this area.

Variable # 15

11. Total V—Total Variability: This measures the amount of variability or inconsistency from one area of self perception to the other. High scores indicate the subject is so variable from one area to another as to reflect little unity or integration.

Variable # 16

12. Column Total V: This score summarizes the variations within columns.

Variable # 17

13. Row Total V: This score is the sum of the variations across the rows.

Variable # 18

14. Distribution Score D: This score measures the degree of certainty as to the way the subject sees himself. High scores mean that the subject is very definite and certain in what he says about himself.

Test IV—Holtzman Ink Blot Test: This is an ink blot test somewhat similar to the Rorschach which delineates personality but is more easily quantifiable. There are 23 "variables" or scores which are obtained. In this study 15 of the 23 were used and each one became a subsequent variable for the cluster analysis.

The Holtzman scores which were employed are as follows:

Variable # 19

1. Space—S: Indicative of oppositional tendencies, resistance or hostility.

Variable #20

2. Color—C: Lack of achromatic or chromatic color is an indication of psychoneurotic tendencies and responsiveness to influences of the environment.

Variable #21

3. Shading—Sh: Excess shading is an indication of intellectualized anxiety, sensitivity and a capacity for warm interpersonal relations.

Variable #22

4. Movement—M: This is an indication of ego strength, developmental maturity and imaginative processes. In excess, high *Ms* indicate fantasy and thought disorder processes.

Variable #23

5. Pathognomic Verbalization—V: This is an indication of psychotic thought processes.

Variable #24

6. Integration—I: This is an indicator of bizarre ideation. It is also an indicator of the degree of seeking relationship between the separate fact of experience and achieving an organized view of the world.

Variable #25

7. Human—H: This is an indicator of a rich inner life, ability to empathize and conscious control over own feelings and impulses.

Variable #26

8. Animal—A: Large number of animal responses indicate aggression and the coming to the fore of basic instincts.

Variable #27

9. Anatomy—At: This indicates a narcissistic preoccupation with self and in some instances, depending on the anatomical responses, schizophrenic tendencies.

Variable #28

10. Sex—Sx (Sex responses): In some cases, a large

number of sex responses is also an indicator of pathological thinking.

Variable #29

11. Abstract—Ab: This is an indication of over-intellectualization, and depending upon the relationship with other variables, high scores indicate significant psychopathology.

Variable #30

12. Anxiety—Ax: Here anxiety indicates such emotions as fear sorrow, and pity.

Variable #31

13. Hostility—Hs: Indicates tendencies which are destructive or potentially destructive toward man.

Variable #32

14. Balance—B: This is also an indication of psychotic ideation.

Variable #33

15. Popular—P: This is an indication of ties to reality. High scores indicate good ties to reality.

EXPERIMENTAL RESULTS

These factors were extracted from the data as a result of the cluster analysis. The definitions of these factors are as follows:

Factor I

*Test and Scale**	*Definition*
1. Total I—Tennessee Self Concept Scale:	Self Worth in General
2. R2—Tennessee Self Concept Scale:	Self Satisfaction and Self Acceptance
3. R3—Tennessee Self Concept Scale:	Perception of Own Behavior

*see list of variables and variable number above.

4. CA—Tennessee Self Concept Scale: Perception of physical self including body, state of health, physical appearance and sexuality.
5. CB—Tennessee Self Concept Scale: Perception of Moral and Ethical Self.
6. CC—Tennessee Self Concept Scale: Perception of personal worth including feeling of adequacy as a person and evaluation of his personality.
7. CD—Tennessee Self Concept Scale: Perception of social self including adequacy and worth in his social interaction with other people in general.

This factor was tentatively named physical, moral, social, personal self concept and self worth, self acceptance and self satisfaction in general.

Factor II

1. Pathognomic Verbalization—Holtzman: Psychotic Thought
2. Sex—Holtzman: Sexual Dysfunction and Pathological Thinking
3. Abstract—Holtzman: Over intellectualization
4. Anxiety—Holtzman: Evidence of fear and sorrow.

Factor III

This factor encompassed the 3 scales of the Multiple Affect Check List and two of the Holtzman—movement and human. The galaxy of words that would describe this factor would be fearful, discouraged and angry with possible thought disorder. This factor is indicative of psychopathology but to a much lesser extent than Factor II.

In order to determine the "strength" of each cardiac group on each factor, the mean T scores were computed on each factor for each cardiac group. Results are shown on the accompanying graph (Figure I).

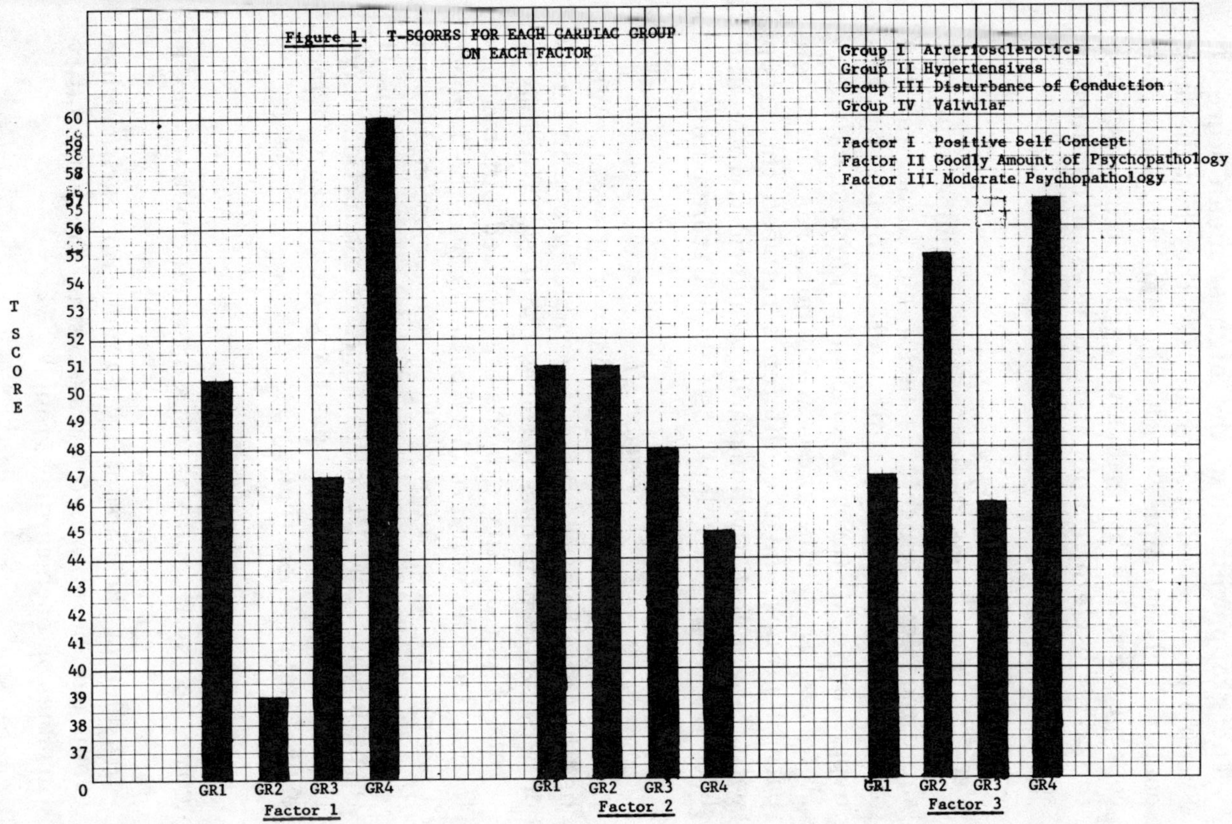

Figure 1. T-SCORES FOR EACH CARDIAC GROUP ON EACH FACTOR

Factor I

The group which had the highest mean score on Factor I was the valvular group, i.e., they had the most positive self concept. Those who had the worst self concept were the hypertensive cardiac patients, with the arteriosclerotic and disturbances of conduction somewhere in between.

Factor II

The group which had the greatest psychopathology in the dimensions which this factor measured was the arteriosclerotic group followed in order by the hypertensive, disturbance of conduction and valvular. However, the differences were not great between patient groups and the difference between the group with the greatest psychopathology (arteriosclerotic) and least pathology (valvular) was only 6 T-score points.

Factor III

On Factor III, we see a peculiar set of events. What had hitherto been the most "favorable" group in terms of personality dynamics becomes the least favorable in terms of personality dimensions spelled out by this factor. The valvular group of patients had the highest T score and were followed by the arteriosclerotic and disturbance of conduction. Thus, patient groups II (hypertensive) and III (disturbance of conduction) have approximately the same positions on the two factors expressing psychopathology.

COMPARISON OF EACH VARIABLE ON EACH CARDIAC GROUP

An idea of the personality dynamics of each cardiac group can be obtained by assessing the personality variables on each cardiac group.

Arteriosclerotic Heart Diseases

The six highest variables in descending order in this cardiac group are anatomy, sex, abstract, total V (2), and color—suggesting a narcisstic preoccupation with self, lack of integration in self concept and pathological thinking. Perusing Figure I, cardiac group I is highest on Factor II, reinforcing the results of these variables on this cardiac group. These patients do have a large amount of psychopathology, since this group consists of patients who have coronary artery disease. Implications for physicians who treat the patients as well as what these patients must look out for by themselves will be given later on.

Hypertensive Vascular Disease

The highest variables in descending order in this group of heart patients was self criticism, distribution, and popular—all positive personality attributes; and three which are negative personality variables—anxiety, movement and hostility. Evidently there is an element of psychopathology in these patients involving anxiety and hostility, two of the variables making up the Multiple Affect Check List.

Disturbance of Conduction

The highest variables in this group in descending order are human, space, row total, column total, popular and movement. This group has a large amount of psychopathology involving oppositional tendencies, a very rich inner life, little unity or integration in self concept, and a rich fantasy life. These patients are in good contact with reality.

Valvular Patients

These are undoubtedly the best adjusted and best integrated of all the heart patients. The highest variables in descending order are Column D, Total P, Row P, Column E, Column B, and Row_3P indicating high self concept and worth in self as family person, worth in general, social self, moral-ethical self and perception of self as functioning and behaving in a positive manner.

A special note should be made on the results of the Cardiac Adjustment Scale. This scale, as noted previously, determines the readiness of patients for safe return to work. Scores of 136 and above are considered well adjusted; scores of 116-135 moderately adjusted; and scores of 0-115 poorly adjusted. The mean score of persons who have a variety of different kinds of heart disease (arteriosclerotic, rheumatic hypertensives and miscellaneous) who are currently gainfully employed at least on a half time basis as described in the Manual of the Cardiac Adjustment Scale was 132 (percentile equivalent of 67); for those who were not working it was 121 (percentile score of 37). In order to get an idea of whether the patients in this study were able to get back to work or not, the median percentile score for each group was computed and then each group ranked as to ability to return to work.

Rank #	Patient Group	Median	Score
1.	Valvular	119	28
2.	Arteriosclerotic	113	23
3.	Disturbance of Conduction	108	17
4.	Hypertensive	81	3

Thus, although the valvular group had the highest priority of all the heart patients in this study insofar as going back to work was concerned, none of the disease entities studied were actually eligible, according to this test. This, in fact, was the case, and very few of these heart patients were working at the time of the study. The significance of this fact insofar as physicians are concerned will be discussed later.

Chapter Six

SUGGESTIONS FOR PHYSICIANS AND PATIENTS

History taking is important in diagnosis and treatment in all areas of medicine, but it is especially so of cardiac diseases. The following are suggestions for physicians in the diagnosis and treatment of the cardiac diseases and their subgroups studied in this project, as well as suggestions to patients who are afflicted. I would stress the importance of *every* cardiac patient heeding the advice of his physician under all circumstances.

Arteriosclerotic Heart Disease

In the group of heart patients studied here, there were the following subgroups: angina pectoris (also considered by many a symptom), myocardial infarction, coronary artery disease, atherosclerosis. In the taking of histories of patients suspected of having arteriosclerotic heart disease or any of the above subgroups, in addition to the usual clinical and medical history, physicians should be careful to get a complete family history, particularly whether the mother or anyone in the mother's family had heart disease. Since this type of cardiac patient did show a large amount of psychopathology, a rather extensive psychological and psychiatric history should be taken both of the patient and the patient's family, with particular reference to the extent to which they are preoccupied with their ailment and what they think of themselves. The whole area of self concept should be explored with specific reference to the moral, ethical, physical and intellectual selves. Past psychiatric history should be elicited since these patients were highest on Factor II, the factor with the greatest psychopathology. Particular attention should be paid to narcissistic preoccupation with the body organs, particularly the heart. Sexual anomalies and bizarre thinking should be carefully observed. Since tremors and temper tantrums seemed to be prevalent in this group, questions about these characteristics should be asked. Exercise has been a controversial element concerning both the cause and treatment of arteriosclerotic heart diseases. However, in the patients studied here, exercise seemed to exacerbate the symptoms. The type, intensity, duration and frequency of exercise should be carefully considered for each patient, and certainly highly competitive athletics demanding sudden or extended bursts of energy should not be encouraged. A moderate climate may not be only a physiological but also a psychological therapeutic agent since these patients said that adverse weather conditions did make their symptoms worse. In general, these patients should avoid alcohol and fatty foods. Although the results are not incontrovertible, if possible, they should not smoke. The advice offered by Rosenman and Friedman on type A Cardiac patients (coronary) on avoiding "hurry sickness" should be heeded. If a patient with arteriosclerotic heart disease has a psychological or psychiatric problem, referral to a psychiatrist or clinical psychologist should be made since what might seem a mild psychological problem may be an indication of deeper underlying psychopathology.

For those of you who have arteriosclerotic heart disease, the cardinal rule is to heed the advice of your physician. The previous suggestions given to the physicians should "be taken to heart", i.e., no fatty foods or alcohol, and if possible do not smoke. Do not hesitate to get professional help in the psychiatric area but only if you think you need it. Slow down the pace of your life and exercise only under the direction of your physician.

Hyptertensive Vascular Disease

It is rather interesting that although the hypertensive group subjectively said they had a high regard for themselves, they were lowest on Factor I, the general self concept factor. Thus, these patients may put up "a good front" and physicians should be alerted to the possibility that this may mask a poor self concept. Like arteriosclerotics, hypertensives encompass a large amount of Type A personality, and these cardiac patients also should avoid "hurry sickness". Physicians examining or taking histories of patients suspected of having hypertensive vascular disease should question them about the headaches—currently and as a child. Information about temper tantrums as a child, and tremors as an adult and as a child should be elicited. Periods of intellectualized and free floating* anxiety seem to be components of the personality of these patients and physicians should carefully ascertain when these periods occur and what happens during these periods. Irascibility and withdrawal from difficult situations are pathognomoic of the hypertensives. The kind of things which make the patient angry and the kind of situations the patient withdraws from should be elicited. Psychotherapy may

*In intellectuatized anxiety the cause is known; in free floating anxiety the cause is not known.

go a long way toward alleviating some of the psychological problems of these patients. Psychotherapy should be oriented to improving self concept. Relief from anxiety and hostility should be an important therapeutic goal for this cardiac group.

Disturbance of Conduction

Disturbance of Conduction may be a component of other kinds of heart disease, and in and of itself may be the most frightening symptom of all the different kinds of heart disease. Thus, this aspect of the ailment may be an important contributing factor to the dynamics found.

Physicians should carefully elicit the family history of these patients insofar as incidence of heart disease is concerned. In this history, the incidence of the patient's headaches, temper tantrums and tremors as a child and adult also should be obtained. A work history with particular reference to how well the patient got along with his (her) boss and co-workers is helpful. The physician should note elements of hostility and oppositional tendencies and also be on the lookout for introversive tendencies and fantasies. He should also be aware that this disease can be very frightening to the patient, and he must allay this fear by providing an accurate, supportive description with a clear prognosis. Mood swings should be carefully observed and an attempt should be made to keep the patient on an "even keel". Alcohol and fatty foods should be consumed sparingly and probably be eliminated from the diet altogether.

For those who have a disturbance of conduction, eliminate alcohol and fatty foods. When you see yourself about to get angry, use the old technique of counting to 10. You must "take it easy". If you see your anger getting out of bounds at times, do not hesitate to get professional help. Slow down the pace of your life. If you feel that your heart is beating irregularly, consult your physician immediately, but do not get unduly frightened since this is an integral part of your illness which under medical supervision should go away. Try to avoid emotional stress.

Valvular Disease

Undoubtedly the valvular patients as a whole are the best adjusted, have the least psychopathology, are the best integrated and have the best self concept of all the groups. It may be that among all the various kinds of heart disease, psychological influences play the least part in the *etiology* of the various valvular problems. These problems are primarily organic in origin (rheumatic, subacute bacterial endocardetis, trauma, congenital syphilis, etc.). Another factor is that the prognosis and outlook for people with valvular diseases has been markedly improved with the advent of modern heart and vascular surgery. However, a person with any kind of valvular disease should restrict his smoking or stop altogether, and eliminate fatty foods and alcohol.

A FINAL WORD

Any kind of heart ailment is, of course, a serious problem not only to the patient and his physician but to people around him. Much is now known about genetics and its influence on the etiology of heart disease. It is known (borne out by the results of this project) that there is a familial diathesis in certain kinds of heart disease. However, as of the writing of this book, no one knows the *precise* influence of genetic and environmental factors in the etiology and pathology of any of the various kinds of heart disease. However, we do know that the genetic influence is more important and occurs more often in certain kinds of cardiac involvement than others (e.g., in arteriosclerotic heart disease). Research in the area of endocrine functioning is also an important element in etiology but endocrinologists still do not know, for example, precisely what role rennin plays in the pathology of heart ailments. Of course, prevention and etiology are intertwined and by knowing the personality attributes of different kinds of heart patients as well as their dietary, smoking, alcohol, and exercise habits, we can suggest steps for both patient and physician which will prevent many cardiac problems. I hope this book will prove to be one of the first steps in achieving this end.

BIBLIOGRAPHY

1. Selzer, A. *The Heart, Its Function in Health and Disease*. Berkeley, California: University of California Press, 1966, p. 88.
2. Selzer, A. ibid, p. 183.
3. Freud, S. *Collected Papers–Vol*. I. New York: International University Press, 1924, p. 76.
4. Wendkos, M. S. "The Influence of Autonomic Imbalance on the Human Electrocardiogram," *American Heart Journal,* 28, 1944, p. 549.
5. Wolf, G. A. Jr. and Wolff, H. G. "Studies on the Nature of Certain Symptoms Associated with Cardiovascular Disorders," *Psychosomatic Medicine,* 8, 1946, pp. 293-319.
6. Hickam, J. B., Cargill, W.H., and Golden, A. "Cardiovascular Reactions to Emotional Stimuli, Effect on the Cardiac Output, Arteriovenous Oxygen Difference, Arterial Pressure and Peripheral Resistance," *J. Clinical Investigation,* 27, 1948, p. 290.
7. Dunbar, F. *Psychosomatic Medicine*. New York: Hoeber, 1943.
8. Arlow, J. "Identification Mechanisms in Coronary Occlusion," *Psychosomatic Medicine*, 7, 1945, p. 195.
9. Miles, H. H. W., Waldfogel, S., Barrabbee, E. L., and Cobb, S. "Psychosomatic Study of 46 Young Men with Coronary Artery Disease," *Psychosomatic Medicine,* 16, 1954, pp. 455-477.
10. Gildea, E. F. "Special Features of Personality
11. White, Paul D. "Psyche and Soma—Spiritual and
12. Kemple, C. "Rorschach Method and Psychosomatic Personality Traits of Patients with Rheumatic Disease, Hypertensive Vascular Disease, Coronary

Occlusion and Fracture," *Psychosomatic Medicine,* 7, 1945, pp. 85-89.

13. Geist, H. *Psychological Aspects of Rheumatoid Arthritis.* Springfield, Illinois: C. C. Thomas & Co., 1966.
14. Gressel, G. C., Shobe, F. O., Saslow, G., Dubois, P. M., and Schroeder H. A. "Personality Factors in Arterial Hypertension," *J.A.M.A.,* 140, 1949, pp. 265-272.
15. Rennie, T.A.C. "The Role of Personality in Certain Hypertensive States," *New England Journal of Medicine,* 221, 1939, pp. 448-456.
16. Friedman, M. and Rosenman, R. H. "Overt Behavior Pattern in Coronary Artery Disease with Blood and Cardiovascular Findings," *J.A.M.A.,* 169, 1959, p. 1286.
17. Rosenman, R. H. et al. "A Predictive Study of Coronary Heart Disease," *J.A.M.A.,* 189, 1964, pp. 15-22.
18. Ginsparb, S. L. and Satten, S. "Psychiatric Aspects of Rehabilitation in Coronary Artery Disease," Proceeding of the 78 Annual Convention of the American Psychological Association, 1970.
19. Gentry, W. D., Foster, S., and Haney, T. "Denial as a Determinant of Anxiety and Perceived Health Status in a Coronary Care Unit," *Psychosomatic Medicine,* 34, 1, Jan.-Feb. 1972, pp. 39-44.
20. Cleveland, S. E. and Johnson, D. L. "Personality Patterns in Young Males with Coronary Disease," *Psychosomatic Medicine,* 1962, 24, pp. 600-610.
21. Weiss, E., Dlin, R., Rollin, H. R., Fisher, H. R. and Bepler, C. R. "Emotional Factors in Coronary Occlusion," *A.M.A. Arch. Int. Med.,* 99, 1957, pp. 628-641.

22. Forssman, O. and Lindegård, B. "The Post Coronary Patient—A Multidisciplinary Investigation of Middle Aged Swedish Males," *J. Psychosom. Research,* 3, 1958, p. 89.
23. Ibrahim, M. A. et al. "Personality Traits and Coronary Heart Disease: Utilization of a Cross Sectional Study Designed to Test whether a Psychological Profile Precedes or Follows Manifest Coronary Heart Disease," *J. Chronic Dis.,* 19, 1966, pp. 255-271.
24. Toor, M., Katschalsky, A., Agmon, J., Alkalouf, D. "Atherosclerosis and Related Factors in Immigrants to Israel," *Circulation,* 22, 1960, pp. 265-279.
25. Hinkle, A. et al. "Occupation, Education, and Coronary Heart Disease," *Science,* 161, 1968, pp. 238-245.
26. Kasanen, A., et al. The Significance of Psychic and Socio-economic Stress and other Modes of Life in the Etiology of Myocardial Infarction," *Annals Med. Intern. Fenn.* 52: suppl. 43, 1963.
27. Syme, S. L., et al. "Some Social and Cultural Factors Associated with Occurrence of Coronary Heart Disease," *J. Chron. Dis.* 17, 1964, pp. 277-289.
28. Rahe, R. H., and Paasikivi, J. "Psychosocial Factors and Myocardial Infarction," *J. Psychosomatic Research,* 15, 1971, p. 33.
29. Van der Valk, J. M., and Groen, J. S. "Personality Structure and Conflict Situation in Patients with Myocardial Infarction," *J. Psychosomatic Research,* 11, 1967, p. 41.
30. Parkes, C. M. et al. "Broken Heart: A Statistical Study of Increased Mortality Among Widowers," *Brit. Med., J.,* 1, 1969, p. 740.
31. Wardwell, W. I., Hyman, M., Bahnson, C. B.

"Socio-environmental Antecedants to Coronary Heart Disease in 87 White Males," *Soc. Sci. and Med.,* 2, 1968, p. 165.

32. Shekelle, R. B., Ostfeld, A. M., Paul, O. "Social Status and Incidence of Coronary Heart Disease," *J. Chron. Dis.,* 22, 1969, pp. 381-394.
33. Theorell, T., Linde, E., Fronberg, S., Karlsson, C. and Levi, L. "A Longitudinal Study of 21 Subjects with Coronary Heart Disease—Report #24," From Laboratory for Clinical Stress Research, Stockholm, Nov. 1971.
34. Friedman, M. and Rosenman, R. M. "Comparison of Fat Intake of American Men and Women—Possible Relationship to Incidence of Clinical Coronary Artery Disease," *Circulation,* 16, 1957, pp. 333-347.
35. Jick, H. and Slone, D. et al. "Boston Collaborative Drug Surveillance Program," *Lancet,* II, 1972, pp. 1278-1271.
36. Jick, H. and Slone, D. et al. "Coffee and Myocardial Infarction," *New England Journal of Medicine,* 289, 1973, pp. 63-67.
37. Framingham Study, Kannell, W. B., Dawber, T. R., ibid #34, p. 100.
38. Heyden, S. Unpublished Data.
39. Paul, O. "Stimulants and Coronaries," *Post-graduate Medicine,* 44, 1968, pp. 196-199.
40. Wilhelmin, L. and Tribben. Unpublished Study.
41. Stine, L. A. "Brief Psychotherapy of Psychiatric Reactions to Physical Illness, The Medical Patient," in *The Psychology of Medical Practice,* Marc H. Hollender, Editor. W. B. Saunders, 1958, pp. 35-59.

APPENDIX I

HEART DISEASE QUESTIONNAIRE

(To be administered by Psychologist. Not to be administered by patient directly.)

Diagnosis ______

Medication ______

Name ______ Address ______ Telephone ______ Age ______

Marital Status __M__ __S__ __W__ __D__ ______ Anyone else in family have heart disease?

Date first notice symptoms ______ What were they? ______

At That Time

a. Anything unusual happening psychologically such as:

1. Mental stress or upset emotionally due to:

a. Loss of someone close to you? ______ If so, what relation? ______
b. Difficulty with career or money? ______
c. Other? ______

To What Extent Do You Think You Are Disabled?:

1. Severely Disabled ______ 2. Moderately Disabled ______ 3. Not Disabled ______

What is the reaction of your relatives, friends, or acquaintances to your heart trouble:

	Indifferent	Greatly Upset	Moderately Upset	Mildly Upset	Other
Relatives	______	______	______	______	______
Friends	______	______	______	______	______
Acquaintances	______	______	______	______	______

Have you lost anyone (by death, moving, etc.) close to you before or after symptoms?

______ Father ______ Mother ______ Other Blood Relative ______ Other Person (Relationship) ______ None

If so, what were the changes in the symptoms? ______

HEART DISEASE QUESTIONNAIRE - 2

As a child or adult, did you or do you have: (Please circle appropriate number)

1. Very Often (Every Day)
2. Quite Often (Once every three days)
3. Moderately Often (Between one a week and one a month)
4. Hardly Ever (Once a month or less)
5. Never

	Child	Adult
Headaches	1 2 3 4 5	1 2 3 4 5
Tremors	1 2 3 4 5	1 2 3 4 5
Tics	1 2 3 4 5	1 2 3 4 5
Convulsions	1 2 3 4 5	1 2 3 4 5
Enuresis (Bedwetting after 4 years of age)	1 2 3 4 5	1 2 3 4 5
Temper Tantrums	1 2 3 4 5	1 2 3 4 5
Stuttering	1 2 3 4 5	1 2 3 4 5
Heart Pains	1 2 3 4 5	1 2 3 4 5
Bite Nails	1 2 3 4 5	1 2 3 4 5
Suck Thumb	1 2 3 4 5	1 2 3 4 5

Do you get angry easily? ______ Yes ______ No

Do you withdraw from difficult situations? ______ Yes ______ No

Ifso, explain: ____

Comments ____

Do you consider yourself:	Yes	No
1. An ambitious person	___	___
2. A persistent person	___	___
3. Have good control of yourself	___	___
4. A moody person	___	___
If yes, explain when you have change in moods ____________________		
5. A clean person	___	___

6. A dependent independent adequate inadequate person (circle)

7. Are you able to express your feelings adequately or do you repress them?

Expression of: Grief ______ Able ______ Unable   Joy ______ Able ______ Unable

Rage ______ Able ______ Unable   Other emotions ______ Able ______ Unable

HEART DISEASE QUESTIONNAIRE - 3

8. Do you conform most of the time to everyday mores? ________ Yes ________ No

9. Do you dream at all? ________

Frequency: Practically every night ____ Once every few nights ____ One night per week ____ Less than one night per week ____

Vividness: Very clear ____ Moderately Clear ____ Jumbled Up ____

Duration: All night ____ Half the night ____ Less than 1/2 night ____

10. Do you daydream? ________

Frequency: Practically every day ____ Once every few days ____ One day per week ____ Less than one day per week ____

Vividness: Very Clear ____ Moderately Clear ____ Jumbled Up ____

What about? ________________________________

11. In relation to your family, describe:

a. Mother's personality and how you got along with her ________________
b. Father's personality and how you got along with him ________________
c. Siblings' personality and how you got along with them ________________

____

12. In your home when you were growing up:

a. Who was disciplinarian: ____ Father ____ Mother ____ Other person, relationship

13. What is the feeling in your family about heart disease? ________________

14. Do you or did any members of your family have any psychosomatic ailments, that is, sicknesses which have no apparent physical cause? ________

If yes: ____ Mother ____ Father ____ Other blood relative, relationship ____ None

15. Work History: Current employment or last job ________________ How Long? ________
Dates ________ Enjoy current work or last job? ________ How getting along with boss or got along with boss? ____ good ____ fair ____ badly Other employees ____ good ____ fair ____ badly
Past work ________________ Type ____ None How got along with boss ____ good ____ fair ____ badly
Other employees ____ good ____ fair ____ badly

HEART DISEASE QUESTIONNAIRE - 4

16. Have you strong religious beliefs?

    1. Extremely religious (go to place of worship regularly and observe all religious holidays) ______
    2. Moderately religious (go to place of worship occasionally and observe some holidays) ______
    3. Rarely go to place of worship ______
    4. Never go to place of worship and never observe holidays ______

17. How much did you indulge in the following previous to heart condition?

    a. Alcohol

    1. Great deal (get inebriated more than once a week) ______
    2. Moderate (get inebriated once a week) ______
    3. Rarely (less than once a week) ______

    b. Smoking

    1. More than one pack a day ______
    2. About one pack a day ______
    3. Less than one pack a day ______
    4. Do not smoke ______

    c. Drugs (exclusive of medication)

    1. Indicate kind and method of taking ______ Kind

       ______ Oral ______ Intravenous ______ Other, describe

       Intake: ______ every day ______ once every few days ______ once per week ______ once every two weeks

       ______ once a month ______ once every few months

    2. None ______

    d. Exercise ______ great deal ______ moderate ______ mild ______ never

    e. Fatty foods ______ great deal ______ moderate ______ small amount ______ never

18. How do you feel about the doctor examining you: ______ good ______ doesn't bother me ______ resist it

19. Are you satisfied with the treatment you are getting? ______ yes ______ no

Comment: ______________________________

____

20. Are your symptoms increased

	Yes	No	If yes, when
a. When you are emotionally upset?	___	___	___________
b. When you exercise?	___	___	___________
c. Under certain weather conditions?	___	___	___________
d. At certain seasons?	___	___	___________

e. Other times - Specify ______________________________________

____

APPENDIX II

TABLE 2

VARIABLE	ARTERIOSCLEROTIC M	ARTERIOSCLEROTIC F	HYPERTENSIVE M	HYPERTENSIVE F	VALVULAR M	VALVULAR F	DISTURBANCE OF CONDUCTION M	DISTURBANCE OF CONDUCTION F
Age Average	58.65	58.92	55	53.7	43.13	40.5	60	62.5
Sex (%)	59	41	40	60	57	43	67	33

VARIABLE	ARTERIOSCLEROTIC	HYPERTENSIVE	VALVULAR	DISTURBANCE OF CONDUCTION
Marital Status (%)				
Divorced	15	20	14	17
Married	30	0	29	17
Widowed	37	20	7	0
Separated	7	20	36	17
Single	11	40	14	50
Anyone else in family have heart disease (%)				
Father	18	0	5	14
Mother	15	0	22	0
Brother	9	0	11	14
Grandmother	6	0	0	0
Sister	3	0	6	0
Daughter	3	0	0	0
Grandfather	0	0	0	14
Son	0	0	0	14
Wife	0	0	6	0

VARIABLE	ARTERIOSCLEROTIC	HYPERTENSIVE	VALVULAR	DISTURBANCE OF CONDUCTION
Length of time had heart disease (%)				
Under two years	14	0	29	20
Over two years	86	100	71	80
Stress due to: (%)				
Loss of someone close	17	20	21	17
Difficulty with money	10	0	21	33
Other	0	0	0	0
Extent Disabled (%)				
Severely	45	40	14	33
Moderately	52	60	71	50
Not	3	0	14	17
Reaction of relatives (%)				
Indifferent	15	25	23	0
Greatly Upset	38	0	23	33
Moderately Upset	27	75	46	67
Mildly Upset	8	0	8	0
Other	12	0	0	0
Reaction of friends (%)				
Indifferent	24	0	21	0
Greatly Upset	24	0	21	20
Moderately Upset	36	100	43	80
Mildly Upset	4	0	7	0
Other	12	0	7	0

VARIABLE	ARTERIOSCLEROTIC		HYPERTENSIVE		VALVULAR		DISTURBANCE OF CONDUCTION	
Reaction of acquaintances (%)								
Indifferent	36		0		18		0	
Greatly Upset	16		0		27		20	
Moderately Upset	28		75		27		80	
Mildly Upset	4		25		18		0	
Other	16		0		9		0	
Headaches (%)	Child	Adult	Ch.	Ad.	Ch.	Ad.	Child	Adult
Very Often	4	16	0	0	0	0	0	0
Quite Often	0	16	60	20	14	21	0	20
Moderately Often	15	7	0	80	7	14	17	40
Hardly Ever	19	38	0	0	21	50	0	20
Never	62	23	40	0	57	14	83	20
Tremors (%)								
Very Often	0	4	0	0	0	0	0	17
Quite Often	4	0	0	0	0	0	0	0
Moderately Often	0	15	20	20	7	7	0	17
Hardly Ever	12	12	0	20	0	21	17	0
Never	85	69	80	60	93	71	83	67
Tics (%)								
Very Often	0	0	0	0	0	0	0	0
Quite Often	4	4	0	0	0	0	0	0
Moderately Often	0	8	0	0	0	7	0	20
Hardly Ever	8	8	0	0	0	14	0	0
Never	88	80	100	100	100	79	100	80

VARIABLE	ARTERIOSCLEROTIC		HYPERTENSIVE		VALVULAR		DISTURBANCE OF CONDUCTION	
	Child	Adult	Ch.	Ad.	Ch.	Ad.	Child	Adult
Convulsion (%)								
Very often	0	0	0	0	0	0	0	0
Quite often	0	0	0	0	7	0	0	0
Moderately often	4	0	0	0	7	0	0	0
Hardly ever	8	0	0	0	0	7	0	17
Never	88	100	100	100	86	93	100	83
Enuresis (%)								
Very often	0	0	0	0	0	0	0	0
Quite often	0	0	0	0	0	0	0	0
Moderately often	4	0	0	0	0	0	0	17
Hardly ever	0	4	0	0	7	7	33	0
Never	96	96	100	100	93	93	67	83
Temper Tantrum (%)								
Very often	0	0	0	0	0	0	0	0
Quite often	0	4	20	20	7	0	0	0
Moderately often	12	4	20	0	14	7	67	33
Hardly ever	15	12	0	0	14	21	0	17
Never	73	81	60	80	64	71	33	50
Stuttering (%)								
Very often	4	0	0	0	0	0	0	0
Quite often	4	0	0	0	14	7	0	0
Moderately often	0	4	0	0	0	14	0	0
Hardly ever	12	4	0	0	7	21	0	0
Never	80	92	100	100	79	57	100	100

VARIABLE	ARTERIOSCLEROTIC		HYPERTENSIVE		VALVULAR		DISTURBANCE OF CONDUCTION	
Heart Pains (%)	Child	Adult	Ch.	Ad.	Ch.	Ad.	Child	Adult
Very often	0	15	0	0	0	0	17	0
Quite often	0	15	0	0	0	14	0	0
Moderately often	4	27	0	60	7	42	0	17
Hardly ever	12	12	20	40	7	29	0	0
Never	85	31	80	0	86	14	83	83
Bite Nails (%)								
Very often	4	4	0	0	0	0	0	0
Quite often	7	4	0	0	0	8	0	0
Moderately often	7	4	0	0	14	8	17	17
Hardly ever	7	4	0	0	7	0	0	0
Never	74	85	100	100	79	85	83	83
Suck Thumb (%)								
Very often	0	0	0	0	0	0	0	0
Quite often	4	0	0	0	7	0	0	0
Moderately often	7	0	0	0	0	0	17	0
Hardly ever	7	0	0	0	14	0	17	0
Never	81	100	100	100	79	100	67	100
Get Angry Easily (%)	Yes	No	Yes	No	Yes	No	Yes	No
	17	83	60	40	31	69	33	67
Withdraw from difficult situations (%)	Yes	No	Yes	No	Yes	No	Yes	No
	38	62	60	40	43	57	50	50

VARIABLE	ARTERIOSCLEROTIC		HYPERTENSIVE		VALVULAR		DISTURBANCE OF CONDUCTION	
Self-Concept: (%) Consider self	Yes	No	Yes	No	Yes	No	Yes	No
Ambitious	90	10	80	20	71	29	100	0
Persistent	79	21	100	0	92	8	100	0
Good Control of self	100	0	100	0	93	7	83	17
Moody	26	74	80	20	71	29	50	50
Clean	100	0	100	0	100	0	100	0
Dependent		14		20		31		33
Independent		86		80		69		67
Adequate		89		80		86		100
Inadequate		11		20		14		0
Able to express emotions (%)	Able	Unable	A	U	A	U	Able	Unable
Grief	48	52	60	40	46	54	67	33
Joy	93	7	100	0	100	0	83	17
Rage	50	50	60	40	75	25	33	67
Other	87	13	100	0	100	0	60	40
Conform to everyday mores (%)	Yes	No	Yes	No	Yes	No	Yes	No
	96	4	100	0	77	23	100	0

VARIABLE	ARTERIOSCLEROTIC	HYPERTENSIVE	VALVULAR	DISTURBANCE OF CONDUCTION
Dreams: (%)				
Yes	89	100	100	100
No	11	0	0	0
A. Frequency				
Practically all night	8	20	8	33
Once every few nights	36	40	25	33
One night per week	28	40	8	17
Less than one night per week	28	0	58	17
B. Vividness				
Very clear	58	80	42	67
Moderately clear	25	20	42	17
Jumbled	17	0	17	17
C. Duration				
All night	4	0	11	17
Half night	17	0	11	17
Less than half night	78	100	78	67
Daydreams: (%)				
Yes	46	60	38	33
No	54	40	62	67
A. Frequency				
Practically every day	18	100	20	50
Once every few days	27	0	60	0
One day per week	0	0	0	0
Less than one day per week	55	0	20	50

VARIABLE	ARTERIOSCLEROTIC	HYPERTENSIVE	VALVULAR	DISTURBANCE OF CONDUCTION
B. Vividness				
Very clear	56	100	50	100
Moderately clear	44	0	50	0
Jumbled	0	0	0	0
Description of daydreams: (%)				
Vacation	20	0	13	0
Money	20	14	25	0
Work	13	0	13	0
Illness	0	14	0	0
Future	0	14	0	0
Clothes	0	14	0	0
Food	0	14	0	0
Travel	0	14	0	0
Excitement	0	14	0	0
Accomplishments	0	0	0	50
Discipline	0	0	0	50
Other	47	0	50	0
Mother's Personality How one got along with (%)				
Very good	17	0	8	20
Good	65	100	85	60
Fair	9	0	8	20
Poor	9	0	0	0
Father's Personality				
Very good	5	0	10	0
Good	63	100	60	75
Fair	21	0	10	25
Poor	11	0	20	0

VARIABLE	ARTERIOSCLEROTIC	HYPERTENSIVE	VALVULAR	DISTURBANCE OF CONDUCTION
Sibling's Personality (%)				
Very good	0	0	0	0
Good	67	100	77	50
Fair	24	0	23	25
Poor	9	0	0	25
Disciplinarian in Family (%)				
Father	32	50	35	33
Mother	64	50	65	50
Other	4	0	0	17
Feeling in Family about Heart Disease (%)				
Accept	33	25	8	0
Upset	14	0	0	0
Indifferent	29	0	17	17
Don't Know	10	50	25	33
Serious Problem	14	0	25	17
Sympathetic	0	25	25	0
Other	0	0	0	33
Psychosomatic Ailments in Family (%)				
Yes	31	20	33	33
No	69	80	67	67
Mother	33	0	0	33
Father	0	0	0	0
Other	67	100	100	67
Religious Beliefs (%)				
Extremely religious	19	25	31	0
Moderately religious	44	50	23	60
Rarely go to place of worship	26	25	23	40
Never go to place of worship	11	0	23	0

VARIABLE	ARTERIOSCLEROTIC	HYPERTENSIVE	VALVULAR	DISTURBANCE OF CONDUCTION
Average Job Length (years)	10.94	14.25	4.77	2.00
Enjoy Job (%)				
Yes	88	100	73	80
No	0	0	0	20
Other	12	0	27	0
Get along with Boss (%)				
Good	100	100	100	80
Fair	0	0	0	20
Badly	0	0	0	0
Get along with Others (%)				
Good	100	100	100	75
Fair	0	0	0	25
Badly	0	0	0	0
Past Work Get along with Boss (%)				
Good	92	100	100	50
Fair	8	0	0	25
Badly	0	0	0	25
Get along with Others (%)				
Good	100	100	100	50
Fair	0	0	0	50
Badly	0	0	0	0

VARIABLE	ARTERIOSCLEROTIC	HYPERTENSIVE	VALVULAR	DISTURBANCE OF CONDUCTION
Drug Use (%)				
None	69	67	58	100
Anacin	14	17	17	0
Other	17	17	8	0
Illegal (Marijuana, Methedrine)	0	0	8	0
Qualude	0	0	8	0
Method (%)				
Oral	100	100	100	0
Intravenous	0	0	0	0
Other	0	0	0	0
Intake (%)				
Every day	50	100	100	0
Once every few days	0	0	0	0
Once a week	0	0	0	0
Once every two weeks	0	0	0	0
Once a month	0	0	0	0
Once every few months	50	0	0	0
Feelings about Doctor's examination (%)				
Good	70	60	77	50
Doesn't bother me	30	20	23	50
Resist it	0	20	0	0
Satisfaction with treatment (%)				
Yes	93	100	100	100
No	4	0	0	0
Indifferent	4	0	0	0

VARIABLE	ARTERIOSCLEROTIC	HYPERTENSIVE	VALVULAR	DISTURBANCE OF CONDUCTION
Are symptoms increased when:				
A. Emotionally upset (%)				
Yes	37	80	54	83
No	63	20	46	17
B. Exercise (%)				
Yes	65	40	54	50
No	35	60	46	50
C. Weather Conditions (%)				
Yes	46	40	15	33
No	54	60	85	67
D. Certain Seasons (%)				
Yes	42	40	31	33
No	58	60	69	67
E. Other times (%)				
Yes	22	0	0	33
No	78	100	100	67

TOTAL CARDIAC GROUP

VARIABLE	1*	2**	3***	4****
Religion (%)	20	41	27	12
Alcohol (%)	12	29	45	14
Smoking (%)	27	10	31	33
Exercises (%)	16	40	41	4
Fatty Foods (%)	18	35	31	12

	Religion	Alcohol	Smoking	Exercise	Fatty Foods
*	Extremely	Great deal	More than 1 pack/day	Great deal	Great deal
**	Moderately	Moderate	About 1 pack/day	Moderate	Moderate
***	Rarely	Rarely	Less than 1 pack/day	Mild	Small amount
****	Never	Never	Do not smoke	Never	Never

Table No 3

		1 A	2 D1	3 H	4 CAS	5 SC	6 TOT1	7 R1	8 R2
1	A	1.000	.881	.837	.095	-.620	.501	.602	.298
2	D1	.881	1.000	.707	.061	-.591	.325	.607	.097
3	H	.837	.707	1.000	.160	-.515	.413	.452	.263
4	CAS	.095	.061	.160	1.000	-.125	.503	.521	.393
5	SC	-.620	-.591	-.515	-.125	1.000	-.560	-.411	-.407
6	TOT1	.501	.325	.413	.503	-.560	1.000	.609	.901
7	R1	.602	.607	.452	.521	-.411	.609	1.000	.264
8	R2	.298	.097	.263	.393	-.407	.901	.264	1.000
9	R3	.481	.283	.407	.380	-.605	.876	.440	.718
10	CA	.088	0.	.138	.509	-.477	.709	.180	.759
11	CB	.616	.372	.495	.241	-.329	.815	.482	.695
12	CC	.320	.138	.180	.320	-.655	.907	.502	.815
13	CD	.578	.515	.559	.378	-.375	.756	.699	.607
14	CE	.245	.158	.160	.721	-.414	.784	.479	.759
15	TOT2	-.265	-.054	-.328	-.407	.160	-.691	.027	-.811
16	COLTOT	-.249	-.050	-.315	-.246	.407	-.691	.080	-.821
17	ROWTOT	-.096	-.020	-.104	-.465	-.561	-.133	-.122	-.140
18	D3	.044	-.095	-.059	-.035	-.469	.299	-.072	.354
19	SPACE	-.067	.035	-.185	.261	-.401	.347	.668	.083
20	COLOR	-.124	.041	-.117	.242	.305	-.617	-.323	-.512
21	SHADE	.154	.153	-.113	.224	.583	-.429	-.900	.002
22	MOVE	.324	.674	.666	-.069	-.114	-.559	.126	-.675
23	PATHO	-.153	.091	.146	.280	.373	-.052	-.292	.192
24	INTEG	.024	.289	-.043	.285	-.021	-.229	-.418	-.039
25	HUMAN	-.745	-.588	-.545	.155	.104	.269	-.019	.195
26	ANIMAL	.657	.465	-.150	.171	-.576	.384	.288	.363
27	ANATMY	-.236	-.479	-.796	.439	.006	.701	.195	.602
28	SEX	.027	.218	.144	.386	.537	-.286	-.090	-.185
29	ABSTRT	-.388	-.213	-.057	.446	.376	.023	-.341	.304
30	ANXIET	.019	.348	.318	.155	.160	-.201	-.256	-.043
31	HOSTIL	-.144	.128	.119	.179	.032	.089	-.287	.343
32	BALNCE	.061	.206	.144	.290	.350	-.378	-.607	-.043
33	POPLAR	-.227	.156	.507	-.205	.569	-.659	-.427	-.481

CORRELATION MATRIX --- EACH VARIABLE WITH EVERY OTHER VARIABLE

CORRELATION MATRIX

		9 R3	10 CA	11 CB	12 CC	13 CD	14 CE	15 TOT2	16 COLTOT
1	A	.481	.088	.616	.320	.578	.245	-.265	-.249
2	D1	.283	0.	.372	.138	.515	.158	-.054	-.054
3	H	.407	.138	.495	.180	.559	.160	-.328	-.315
4	CAS	.380	.509	.241	.320	.378	.721	-.407	-.246
5	SC	-.605	-.477	-.329	-.655	-.375	-.414	.160	.407
6	TOT1	.876	.709	.815	.907	.756	.784	-.691	-.693
7	R1	.440	.180	.482	.502	.699	.479	.027	.080
8	R2	.718	.759	.695	.815	.607	.759	-.811	-.821
9	R3	1.000	.645	.803	.850	.562	.587	-.700	-.743
10	CA	.645	1.000	.276	.719	.317	.744	-.648	-.781
11	CB	.803	.276	1.000	.674	.628	.482	-.683	-.563
12	CC	.850	.719	.674	1.000	.535	.697	-.513	-.606
13	CD	.562	.317	.628	.535	1.000	.387	-.358	-.335
14	CE	.587	.744	.482	.697	.387	1.000	-.599	-.564
15	TOT2	-.700	-.648	-.683	-.513	-.358	-.599	1.000	.923
16	COLTOT	-.743	-.781	-.563	-.606	-.335	-.564	.923	1.000
17	ROWTOT	-.038	.190	-.424	.121	-.127	-.204	.385	.002
18	D2	.358	.560	-.151	.539	-.320	-.438	-.273	-.435
19	SPACE	.270	.300	-.051	.166	.659	.432	.093	-.026
20	COLOR	-.618	-.238	-.805	-.586	-.103	-.691	.448	.404
21	SHADE	-.482	-.207	-.134	-.497	-.497	-.357	-.354	-.240
22	MOVE	-.552	-.320	-.827	-.445	-.042	-.576	.825	.689
23	PATHO	-.288	.041	-.228	-.127	.286	-.148	-.111	-.009
24	INTEG	-.237	.344	-.695	-.165	-.001	-.290	.060	-.133
25	HUMAN	.514	.529	.046	.328	.182	-.017	-.297	-.345
26	ANIMAL	.185	.056	.354	.555	.028	.482	.080	.030
27	ANATMY	.849	.494	.771	.751	.232	.463	-.595	-.502
28	SEX	-.469	-.436	-.188	-.330	.169	-.417	.243	.464
29	ABSTRT	-.223	.137	-.165	-.085	.314	-.055	-.252	-.153
30	ANXIET	-.313	.195	-.616	-.261	.249	-.261	.074	-.006
31	HOSTIL	-.148	.370	-.346	.053	.327	.049	-.167	-.230
32	BALNCE	-.533	-.221	-.528	-.576	-.031	-.242	-.179	-.205
33	POPLAR	-.719	-.388	-.676	-.732	-.094	-.709	.306	.380

CORRELATION MATRIX

		17 ROWTOT	18 D2	19 SPACE	20 COLOR	21 SHADE	22 MOVE	23 PATHO
1	A	-.096	.044	-.067	-.124	.154	.324	-.153
2	D1	-.020	-.095	.035	.041	.153	.674	.091
3	H	-.104	-.059	-.185	-.117	-.113	.666	.146
4	CAS	.465	-.035	.261	.242	.224	-.069	.280
5	SC	.561	-.469	-.401	.305	.583	-.114	.373
6	TOT1	-.133	.299	.347	-.617	-.429	-.559	-.052
7	R1	-.122	-.072	.668	-.323	-.900	.126	-.292
8	R2	-.140	.354	.083	-.512	.002	-.675	.192
9	R3	-.038	.358	.270	-.618	-.482	-.552	-.288
10	CA	.190	.560	.300	-.238	-.207	-.320	.041
11	CB	-.424	.151	-.051	-.805	-.134	-.827	-.228
12	CC	.121	.539	.166	-.586	-.497	-.445	-.127
13	CD	-.127	-.320	.659	-.103	-.497	-.042	.286
14	CE	-.204	.438	.432	-.691	-.357	-.576	-.148
15	TOT2	.385	-.273	.093	.448	-.354	.825	-.111
16	COLTOT	.002	-.435	-.026	.404	-.240	.689	-.009
17	ROWTOT	1.000	.336	.284	.174	-.316	.444	-.247
18	D2	.336	1.000	-.263	-.555	-.034	-.446	-.470
19	SPACE	.284	-.263	1.000	.050	.220	-.035	-.183
20	COLOR	.174	-.555	.050	1.000	.385	.149	.326
21	SHADE	-.316	-.034	.220	.385	1.000	-.040	.291
22	MOVE	.444	-.446	-.035	.149	-.040	1.000	.448
23	PATHO	-.247	-.470	-.183	.326	.291	.448	1.000
24	INTEG	.445	-.155	.259	.606	.685	.425	.565
25	HUMAN	.059	.052	.513	.139	.183	.079	.160
26	ANIMAL	.125	.510	.114	.096	.489	.198	.177
27	ANATMY	-.308	.409	.108	-.000	.286	-.406	-.022
28	SEX	-.457	-.655	-.107	.335	.371	.377	.788
29	ABSTRT	-.264	-.424	-.177	.435	.286	.073	.847
30	ANXIET	.192	-.480	-.052	.463	.241	.675	.784
31	HOSTIL	.114	-.244	-.020	.320	.259	.524	.903
32	BALNCE	.028	-.405	.187	.708	.774	.112	.414
33	POPLAR	-.118	-.702	-.031	.378	.139	.672	.701

CORRELATION MATRIX

		24 INTEG	25 HUMAN	26 ANIMAL	27 ANATMY	28 SEX	29 ABSTRT	30 ANXIET
1	A	.024	-.745	.657	-.236	.027	-.388	.019
2	D1	.289	-.588	.465	-.479	.218	-.213	.348
3	H	-.043	-.545	-.150	-.796	.144	-.057	.318
4	CAS	.285	.155	.171	.439	.386	.446	.155
5	SC	-.021	.104	-.576	.006	.537	.376	.160
6	TOT1	-.229	.269	.384	.701	-.286	.023	-.201
7	R1	-.418	-.019	.288	.195	-.090	-.341	-.256
8	R2	-.039	.195	.363	.602	-.185	.304	-.043
9	R3	-.237	.514	.185	.849	-.469	-.223	-.313
10	CA	.344	.529	.056	.494	-.436	.137	.195
11	CB	-.695	.046	.354	.771	-.188	-.165	-.616
12	CC	-.165	.328	.555	.751	-.330	-.085	-.261
13	CD	-.001	.182	.028	.232	.169	.314	.249
14	CE	-.290	-.017	.482	.463	-.417	-.055	-.261
15	TOT2	.060	-.297	.080	-.595	.243	-.252	.074
16	COLTOT	-.133	-.345	.030	-.502	.464	-.153	-.006
17	ROWTOT	.445	.059	.125	-.308	-.457	-.264	.192
18	D2	-.155	.052	.510	.409	-.655	-.424	-.480
19	SPACE	.259	.513	.114	.108	-.107	-.177	-.052
20	COLOR	.606	.139	.096	-.000	.335	.435	.463
21	SHADE	.685	.183	.489	.286	.371	.286	.241
22	MOVE	.425	.079	.198	-.406	.377	.073	.675
23	PATHO	.565	.160	.177	-.022	.788	.847	.784
24	INTEG	1.000	.316	.395	.126	.378	.392	.779
25	HUMAN	.316	1.000	.016	.540	.150	.179	.102
26	ANIMAL	.395	.016	1.000	.351	.171	-.027	.152
27	ANATMY	.126	.540	.351	1.000	.039	.078	-.199
28	SEX	.378	.150	.171	.039	1.000	.726	.429
29	ABSTRT	.392	.179	-.027	.078	.726	1.000	.494
30	ANXIET	.779	.102	.152	-.199	.429	.494	1.000
31	HOSTIL	.700	.215	.292	-.055	.503	.674	.893
32	BALNCE	.768	.051	.247	-.050	.286	.468	.549
33	POPLAR	.418	.260	-.134	-.422	.595	.495	.694

CORRELATION MATRIX

		31 HOSTIL	32 BALNCE	33 POPLAR
1	A	-.144	.061	-.227
2	D1	.128	.206	.156
3	H	.119	.144	.507
4	CAS	.179	.290	-.205
5	SC	.032	.350	.569
6	TOT1	.089	-.378	-.659
7	R1	-.287	-.607	-.427
8	R2	.343	-.043	-.481
9	R3	-.148	-.533	-.719
10	CA	.370	.021	-.388
11	CB	-.346	-.528	-.676
12	CC	.053	-.576	-.732
13	CD	.327	-.031	-.094
14	CE	.049	-.242	-.709
15	TOT2	-.167	-.179	.306
16	COLTOT	-.230	-.205	.380
17	ROWTOT	.114	.028	-.118
18	D2	-.244	-.405	-.702
19	SPACE	-.020	.187	-.031
20	COLOR	.320	.708	.378
21	SHADE	.259	.774	.139
22	MOVE	.524	.112	.672
23	PATHO	.903	.414	.701
24	INTEG	.700	.768	.418
25	HUMAN	.215	.051	.260
26	ANIMAL	.292	.247	-.134
27	ANATMY	-.055	-.050	-.422
28	SEX	.503	.286	.595
29	ABSTRT	.674	.468	.495
30	ANXIET	.893	.549	.694
31	HOSTIL	1.000	.465	.639
32	BALNCE	.465	1.000	.360
33	POPLAR	.639	.360	1.000

TABLE NO. 4

VARIABLES IN EACH FACTOR

FACTOR I		FACTOR II		FACTOR III	
Variable Number	Description	Variable Number	Description	Variable Number	Description
6	TOT1	23	PATHO	1	A
8	R2	28	SEX	2	D1
9	R3	29	ABSTRT	3	H
10	CA	30	ANXIET	22	MOVE
11	CB	31	HOSTIL	25	HUMAN
12	CC				
14	CE				

Table No 5

INTERCORRELATION BETWEEN FACTORS

	Factor 1	Factor 2	Factor 3
Factor 1	1.0000	-.1610	.0066
Factor 2	-.1610	1.0000	.1111
Factor 3	.0066	.1111	1.0000

Table No 6

ACCURACY OF FACTOR ESTIMATES

Factor I	.9803
Factor II	.9668
Factor III	.9867

Table No 7

T SCORE MEANS AND SIGMAS OF VARIABLES FOR ASHD GROUP

VARIABLE		MEAN	SIGMA
1	A	47.6173	6.9485
2	D1	47.7882	9.4651
3	H	46.2539	5.1255
4	CAS	49.3654	11.1742
5	SC	51.2347	9.4353
6	TOT1	49.8946	9.3511
7	R1	49.5546	5.7821
8	R2	49.7634	12.0272
9	R3	50.5647	10.0096
10	CA	49.3522	5.5207
11	CB	51.2677	7.3758
12	CC	52.0031	11.0740
13	CD	49.7488	5.7498
14	CE	47.9716	11.5686
15	TOT2	51.9852	11.3002
16	COLTOT	52.6893	11.7649
17	ROWTOT	48.7078	9.3777
18	D2	48.5300	12.2804
19	SPACE	47.4286	7.5377
20	COLOR	51.6524	11.3498
21	SHADE	50.8183	11.2553
22	MOVE	47.5561	8.6398
23	PATHO	51.1379	11.7687
24	INTEG	49.8512	11.2520
25	HUMAN	48.7867	10.2337
26	ANIMAL	51.6757	12.0915
27	ANATMY	54.0724	11.3549
28	SEX	53.7299	11.6872
29	ABSTRT	52.5561	12.3856
30	ANXIET	48.4968	8.7503
31	HOSTIL	49.0187	10.6205
32	BALNCE	49.1390	11.8384
33	POPLAR	47.0033	11.3937

Table No 8

T SCORE MEANS AND SIGMAS OF VARIABLES FOR HYPERTENSIVE VASCULAR GROUP

VARIABLE		MEAN	SIGMA
1	A	53.4227	4.3733
2	D1	54.5441	6.2811
3	H	54.6122	3.6463
4	CAS	42.0939	5.8332
5	SC	59.8773	0.0000
6	TOT1	35.7684	0.0000
7	R1	28.1737	0.0000
8	R2	42.7830	0.0000
9	R3	40.1750	0.0000
10	CA	48.5001	2.9997
11	CB	45.2749	0.0000
12	CC	34.9765	0.0000
13	CD	29.9056	0.0000
14	CE	42.0710	0.0000
15	TOT2	44.8717	0.0000
16	COLTOT	46.0557	0.0000
17	ROWTOT	46.1234	0.0000
18	D2	57.2484	0.0000
19	SPACE	40.0000	0.0000
20	COLOR	46.1119	1.0368
21	SHADE	53.0846	10.5756
22	MOVE	55.1040	11.7787
23	PATHO	51.9117	8.6029
24	INTEG	50.7439	4.4638
25	HUMAN	43.5657	.5147
26	ANIMAL	52.3459	4.0217
27	ANATMY	43.0931	1.5070
28	SEX	45.8463	1.7801
29	ABSTRT	45.4060	0.0000
30	ANXIET	55.5590	13.6990
31	HOSTIL	53.8161	12.2118
32	BALANCE	52.7019	4.9881
33	POPLAR	56.8451	5.2994

Table No 9

T SCORE MEANS AND SIGMAS OF VARIABLES FOR DISTURBANCE OF CONDUCTION GROUP

VARIABLE		MEAN	SIGMA
1	A	43.5193	5.5329
2	D1	47.5447	8.1231
3	H	45.4924	4.0332
4	CAS	49.6665	7.9145
5	SC	50.0000	8.6425
6	TOT1	46.3103	3.5139
7	R1	51.0023	7.2383
8	R2	46.3323	4.1409
9	R3	44.1276	3.9526
10	CA	52.4876	4.2007
11	CB	38.9362	7.4910
12	CC	48.1220	.6260
13	CD	47.4882	5.0236
14	CE	48.5249	2.7659
15	TOT2	56.8654	.4135
16	COLTOT	53.2272	4.4822
17	ROWTOT	60.1222	11.8451
18	D2	54.2071	1.5206
19	SPACE	62.0000	6.0000
20	COLOR	50.5184	4.6706
21	SHADE	45.1528	2.6439
22	MOVE	53.7579	11.7786
23	PATHO	46.8137	2.8677
24	INTEG	52.5294	10.7129
25	HUMAN	63.1259	1.5442
26	ANIMAL	42.6269	1.0055
27	ANATMY	45.7303	1.8837
28	SEX	44.0661	0.0000
29	ABSTRT	47.2194	2.5388
30	ANXIET	50.7941	10.1253
31	HOSTIL	51.5264	5.3426
32	BALNCE	47.7137	7.4822
33	POPLAR	55.5203	1.3248

INDEX